Interpretation of Emergency Head CT

A Practical Handbook

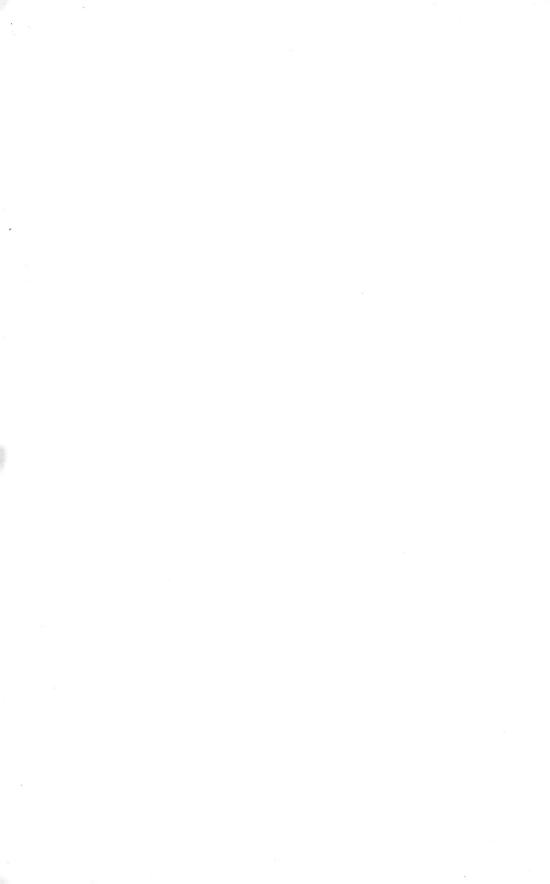

Interpretation of Emergency Head CT

A Practical Handbook

Erskine J. Holmes, MRCS, FCEM
Consultant in Emergency Medicine
Wexham Park Hospital, Slough

Anna C. Forest-Hay, MA, FRCS (A&E) Edin, FCEM
Consultant in Paediatric and Adult Emergency Medicine
Wexham Park Hospital, Slough

Rakesh R. Misra, BSc (Hons), FRCS (Eng), FRCR
Consultant Radiologist, Wycombe Hospital
Buckinghamshire Hospitals NHS Trust

Editor

R. R. Misra

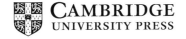

CAMBRIDGE UNIVERSITY PRESS

Cambridge, New York, Melbourne, Madrid, Cape Town, Singapore, São Paulo, Delhi, Dubai, Tokyo

Cambridge University Press
The Edinburgh Building, Cambridge CB2 8RU, UK

Published in the United States of America by Cambridge University Press, New York

www.cambridge.org
Information on this title: www.cambridge.org/9780521682428

First published 2008
Reprinted with corrections 2009

Printed in the United Kingdom at the University Press, Cambridge

A catalogue record for this publication is available from the British Library

ISBN 978-0-521-68242-8 paperback

Cambridge University Press has no responsibility for
the persistence or accuracy of URLs for external or
third-party internet websites referred to in this publication,
and does not guarantee that any content on such
websites is, or will remain, accurate or appropriate.

Every effort has been made in preparing this publication to provide accurate and up-to-date information which is in accord with accepted standards and practice at the time of publication. Although case histories are drawn from actual cases, every effort has been made to disguise the identities of the individuals involved. Nevertheless, the authors, editors and publishers can make no warranties that the information contained herein is totally free from error, not least because clinical standards are constantly changing through research and regulation. The authors, editors and publishers therefore disclaim all liability for direct or consequential damages resulting from the use of material contained in this publication. Readers are strongly advised to pay careful attention to information provided by the manufacturer of any drugs or equipment that they plan to use.

Dedicated to my wife Jill for her support, help and love over the years. **E. J. H.**

I would like to dedicate this book to my father, Iain, for being my inspiration and mentor. **A. F-H.**

Dedicated to my beautiful wife, Rachel, and children, Rohan, Ela and Krishan, for allowing me the time to write this book. **R. R. M.**

CONTENTS

Acknowledgements	*page* ix
Preface	xi
Abbreviations	xii
Introduction	xiii

Section I — 1

Fundamentals of CT imaging	3
History	3
Technical details	4
Windowing and grey scale	6
Tissue characteristics	6
Image artefacts	8
Important anatomical considerations	10
Review of normal anatomy	10
Review of vascular territories	22
Review of vascular anatomy	33

Section 2 — 35

Reviewing a CT scan	36
Acute stroke	38
Ischaemic stroke	38
Haemorrhagic stroke	45
Subdural haematoma (SDH)	50
Extradural haematoma	54
Subarachnoid haemorrhage	58
Cerebral venous sinus thrombosis	62
Contusions	64
Skull fractures	68
Meningitis	71
Raised intracranial pressure	74

Hydrocephalus   77

Abscesses   80

Arteriovenous malformation   83

Solitary lesions   86

Multiple lesions   89

Self-assessment section   92

Self Assessment – Answers   95

Appendices   101

Differential diagnosis of intracerebral lesions   103

CT guidelines for head trauma   105

Proposed algorithm for the emergency management of acute stroke   106

Information required prior to neurosurgical referral   108

ACKNOWLEDGEMENTS

The authors would sincerely like to thank Dr Jagrit Shah, Consultant Radiologist, Queen's Medical Centre, Nottingham, for generously donating several key images.

We would also like to thank Dr Matthew Burn, Consultant Stroke Physician, Wycombe Hospital, Buckinghamshire Hospitals NHS Trust. Matthew read and edited the final manuscript, and provided invaluable advice from a Stroke Physician's perspective. His contribution is greatly appreciated.

Sincere thanks to Luc Bouwman – CT Product Manager, Toshiba Medical Systems, Europe, for meticulously drawing all the superb images in Section 1.

PREFACE

Welcome to the first handbook of CT brain interpretation. Focus has been placed on including a greater number of images than would normally be found in a book of this size. The resolution has been heightened and the accompanying text limited to precise details, in order to achieve our goal: that is to equip a wide variety of medical professionals with a general understanding of head CT. A schema is provided by which to analyse the images, in order to develop greater confidence to diagnose the most common and critical problems. It is hoped that this book will be invaluable to individuals who find themselves, more and more, in the acute decision-making setting. This includes Emergency Physicians, Surgeons, Neurosurgeons, Trauma or Orthopaedic Surgeons, Radiographers and Elderly Care physicians. It is also intended to be instructive to radiology trainees and medical students alike. All choice topics are included, thus lending itself as an excellent revision aid for anyone preparing for a postgraduate exam. Small enough to carry around, we hope we have provided a reliable reference for what you need to remember, regardless of the time of day or night.

ABBREVIATIONS

ACom   Anterior communicating
APTT   Activated partial thromboplastin time
AVM   Arteriovenous malformation
BP   Blood pressure
CCF   Congestive cardiac failure
CSF   Cerebrospinal fluid
CT   Computer tomography
CTV   CT venogram
CVA   Cerebrovascular accident
ECA   External carotid artery
ECG   Electrocardiogram
EDH   Extradural haemorrhage
ETA   Estimated time of arrival
ETT   Endotracheal tube
GCS   Glasgow Coma Scale
HR   Heart rate
HU   Hounsfield Unit
i.m.   intramuscular
INR   International normalised ratio
i.v.   Intravenous
ICA   Internal carotid artery
LP   Lumbar puncture
M:F   Male:female
MCA   Middle cerebral artery
NICE   National Institute of Clinical Excellence
PCom   Posterior communicating
RIND   Reversible ischaemic neurological deficit
RR   Respiratory rate
SAH   Subarachnoid haemorrhage
SDH   Subdural haematoma
SLE   Systemic lupus erythematosus
SSS   Superior sagittal sinus
TIA   Transient ischaemic attack
WCC   White cell count

INTRODUCTION

Computer tomography (CT) is now widely available and is being used more and more, unlike magnetic resonance imaging, 24 hours a day, 7 days a week. CT is often the initial imaging modality of choice; not only for diagnosis but also to guide treatment.

The most common request for CT out of hours is brain imaging. CT is a vital tool in the assessment of patients with serious head injury. It remains the investigation of choice for the assessment of acute haemorrhage and bony injury. Consequently, patient management has been transformed since its inception, as rapid imaging and diagnosis of intracranial pathology can facilitate emergency intervention. Equally, a delay in diagnosis, and treatment, may adversely affect outcome and prognosis.

Patient's expectations of modern medical technology are high. There are ever-increasing time pressures to form rapid diagnoses, and improve efficiency, in the face of a more litigious society. The European Working Time Directive is likely to make doctors feel more vulnerable, with shift patterns reducing personal experience and training opportunities. Furthermore, the multidisciplinary team on duty in the *Hospital at Night Scheme* may not possess the appropriate expertise between them to interpret emergency imaging. Yet, the NICE guidelines are in place to further increase the number of CT scans performed out of hours. To add to this, the nationwide shortage of radiologists results in a limited CT service available out of hours. Hence we have the dilemma of how to provide an adequate emergency imaging service coupled with who will interpret the images.

The College of Emergency Medicine has stipulated that Specialist Registrars in Emergency Medicine are expected to be able to diagnose brain pathology from CT scans of the head. Currently, in many hospitals around the country it is routine for CT head scans, performed out of hours, to be interpreted by the requesting doctor. This is likely to be a progressive future trend, with a variety of speciality groups needing to acquire these skills.

Analogous to this is ECG interpretation; originally the domain of the Cardiologist, this is now a routine general investigation interpreted by most clinicians. It is not inconceivable that medical students, and junior medical staff alike, may need to acquire the basic skills to analyse CT abnormalities in the future, if we are to keep pace with the ever-increasing demand.

The purpose of this book is to provide a systematic approach by which to interpret and *provisionally* report head CT scans, based on learning to recognise common pathologies from an archive of representative images.

SECTION I

Fundamentals of CT imaging

History

- In the early 1970s Sir Godfrey Hounsfield's research produced the first clinically useful CT scans.
- Original scanners took approximately 6 minutes to perform a rotation (one slice) and 20 minutes to reconstruct. Despite many technological advances since then, the principles remain the same.
- On early scanners the tube rotated around a stationary patient with the table then moved to enable a further acquisition. The machine rotated clockwise and counter-clockwise as power was supplied via a cable.
- Modern-day helical or spiral scanners obtain power via slip ring technology, thus allowing continuous tube rotation as the patient moves through the scanner automatically. This allows a volume of data to be acquired in a single rotation, with the benefits of faster scanning, faster patient throughput and less re-imaging as patient movement artefact is reduced.
- New multi-slice scanners use existing helical scanning technology but have multiple rows of detectors to acquire multiple slices per tube rotation. In turn, advanced computer processing power allows reconstructive techniques, such as three-dimensional and multiplanar reformats, to be more easily accessible. Consequently, scans are now performed routinely at a reporting workstation where the image can be viewed dynamically.

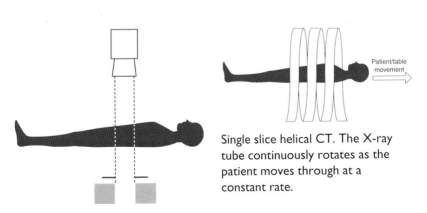

Single slice helical CT. The X-ray tube continuously rotates as the patient moves through at a constant rate.

Single slice system.

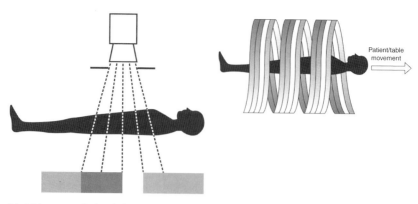

Multidetector helical CT: four detectors shown here.

Technical details

- The X-ray tube produces a narrow fan-shaped beam of collimated X-rays, which pass through the patient to reach a bank of detectors opposite the source.
- X-rays are attenuated differentially by the patient, depending on the tissues through which they pass. Low density tissues such as fat/aerated lung absorb fewer X-rays, allowing more to reach the detector. The opposite is true of dense tissues such as bone.
- The amount of transmitted radiation received provides information on the density of the tissue.
- A CT slice is divided up into a matrix of squares, e.g. 256×256, 512×512 and 1024×1024. The slice thickness determines the volume of these squares; these are called voxels. Using mathematical calculations, the degree to which a tissue absorbs radiation within each voxel, *the linear attenuation coefficient*, μ, is calculated and assigned a value related to the average attenuation of the tissues within it $\equiv$ *the CT number* or *Hounsfield Unit*.
- Each value of μ is assigned a grey scale value on the display monitor and is presented as a square picture element (pixel) on the image.
- Spiral scanners acquire a volume of information from which an axial slice is reconstructed, as above, using computer technology. Slices are created from data during the reconstruction phase.
- *Pitch* is defined as the distance moved by the table in millimetres, during one complete rotation of the X-ray tube, divided by the slice thickness in millimetres. In general, increasing pitch (increase table speed with a fixed slice thickness) reduces radiation dose; as a result image resolution can be affected and thus a compromise usually exists.

$$\text{Pitch} = \frac{\text{Distance moved by the table during one complete rotation}}{\text{Slice thickness}}$$

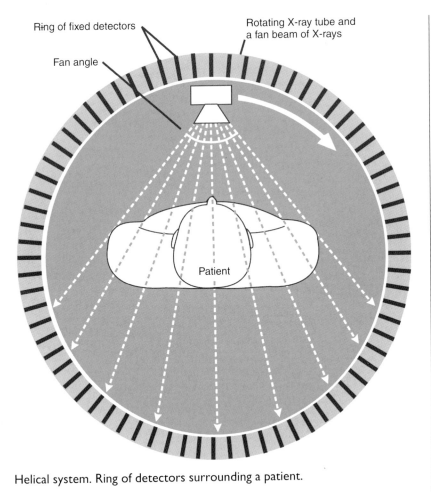

Ring of fixed detectors

Rotating X-ray tube and a fan beam of X-rays

Fan angle

Patient

Helical system. Ring of detectors surrounding a patient.

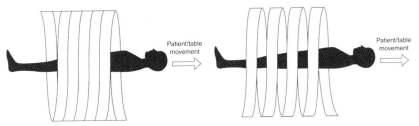

Patient/table movement

Patient/table movement

The pitch is low with the table moving less for each tube revolution, resulting in a sharper image.

The pitch is high, effectively stretching out the helix. The table moves more for each revolution, resulting in some loss of image quality.

Windowing and grey scale

- Modern CT scanners are able to differentiate in excess of 2000 CT numbers; however, the human eye can differentiate only around 30 shades of grey.
- To maximise the perception of medically important features, images can be digitally processed to meet a variety of clinical requirements.
- The grey scale values assigned to processed CT numbers on a display monitor, can be adjusted to suit special application requirements.
- Contrast can be enhanced by assigning just a narrow interval of CT numbers to the entire grey scale on the display monitor. This is called *window technique*; the range of CT numbers displayed on the whole grey scale being called the *window width* and the average value the *window level*.
- Changes in window width alter contrast, and changes in window level select the structures in the image to be displayed on the grey scale, i.e. from black to white.
- Narrowing the window compresses the grey scale to enable better differentiation of tissues within the chosen window. For example, in assessment of CT of the head, a narrow window of approximately 80 HU is used, thus allowing the eye to discriminate tissues only 2–3 HU apart. In practical terms, if we centre the window at 30 HU, then CT numbers above 70 will appear white and those below −10 will appear black. This allows subtle differences in tissue densities to be identified.
- Conversely, if the window is widened to 1500 HU, then each detectable shade of grey would cover 50 HU and soft tissue differentiation would be lost; however bone/soft tissue interfaces would be apparent.
- In practical terms the window width and level are preset on the workstation and can be adjusted by choosing the appropriate setting, i.e. a window setting for brain, posterior fossa, bone, etc.

Tissue characteristics

- Unlike conventional radiography, CT has relatively good contrast resolution and can therefore differentiate between tissues which vary only slightly in density. This is extremely valuable when assessing the brain, as grey and white matter vary only slightly in density.
- Artefacts aside, the densest structure in the head is bone, appearing white on CT. This is followed by acute haematoma, which is denser than flowing blood, due to clot retraction and loss of water. Blood is thought to be hyperdense due to the relative density of the haemoglobin molecule. With time, blood appears isodense and then hypodense, compared to brain parenchyma, due to clot resorption. Rebleeding and layering of blood (haematocrit effect due to gravity) can often cause confusion.

- Brain can be differentiated into grey and white matter due to the difference in fatty myelin content between the two. Typically white matter (higher fatty myelin content – HU ≈ 30) is darker than the adjacent grey matter (HU ≈ 40).
- Fat and air have low attenuation values and can be readily identified.
- CSF has a similar attenuation value to water, appearing black.
- Pathological processes may become apparent due to oedema within, or adjacent to, an abnormality. Oedema is less dense than normal brain.
- Occasionally the use of a contrast medium will reveal an abnormality either due to the inherent vascular nature of a lesion or due to alteration in the normal blood brain barrier.
- Tumours may be very variable in their appearance, but may be hyper-dense due to a high nuclear/cytoplasmic ratio or tumour calcification.

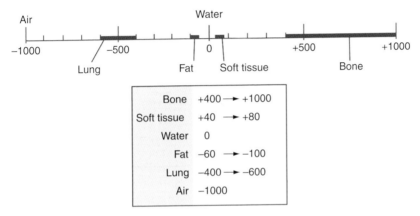

Bone	+400 ⟶ +1000
Soft tissue	+40 ⟶ +80
Water	0
Fat	−60 ⟶ −100
Lung	−400 ⟶ −600
Air	−1000

Hounsfield Scale of CT numbers.

Image artefacts

- An artefact is a visual impression in the image of a feature that does not actually exist in the tissue being imaged. They are important to recognise so as not to be confused with pathology. Artefacts may occur due to scanner malfunction, patient movement and the presence of extrinsic objects within the slice being scanned, e.g. a metal foreign body.
- Fortunately, many artefacts have now been reduced or eliminated by advances in CT speed and technology.
- *Motion artefacts* – Occur with voluntary and involuntary patient motion.
  - Tend to result in streak patterns.
  - Can be reduced by patient co-operation, quicker scan times and software compensation.
- *Partial volume artefacts* – The CT number reflects the average attenuation within the voxel and thus, if a highly attenuating structure is present within the voxel, it will raise the average attenuation value ≡ *partial volume artefact*.
  - Contamination can occur especially with thicker slices and near bony prominences.
  - Always review the slices above and below to assess for structures likely to cause partial volume artefacts.
  - Reduced by using thinner slices (e.g. posterior fossa) and software compensation.
- *Metallic artefacts* – The attenuation coefficient of metal is much greater than any structure within the body. As a result, radiation is completely attenuated by the object and information about adjacent structures is lost.
  - Produces characteristic star-shaped streak artefacts
  - Can be reduced by widening the window; at a cost to intracranial detail.
  - Again, software manipulation may help.
- *Beam hardening artefacts* – Results from an increase in the average energy of the x-ray beam as it passes through a tissue. Think of CT as using a spectrum of radiation energy; low energy radiation is filtered out by high density structures such as bone, leaving higher energy radiation which is less absorbed by soft tissues, thus reducing tissue differentiation.
  - Characterised by linear bands of low attenuation connecting two areas of high density, such as bone, e.g. the posterior fossa.
  - Can be reduced by using a filter to adjust the spectrum of radiation and by post-processing software.

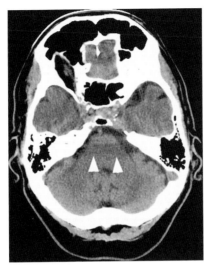

Beam hardening artefact: band of low attenuation across the pons (arrowheads). This reduces tissue differentiation and is characteristic of beam-hardening artefact.

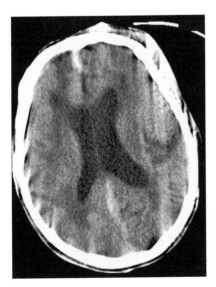

Motion artefact: characteristic movement blurring.

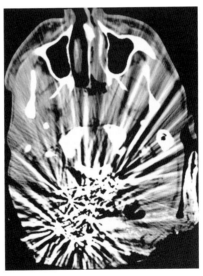

Metallic artefact. Gross star-shaped metallic streaks due to gunshot pellets.

Important anatomical considerations

Review of normal anatomy

Key for cerebral anatomy

1 = Sphenoid sinus
2 = Medulla oblongata
3 = cerebellum

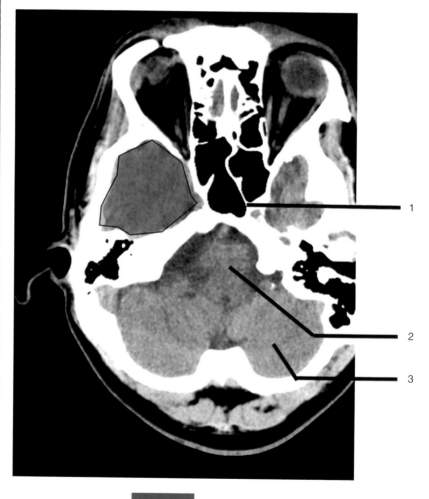

Temporal Lobe

4 = Fourth ventricle
5 = Middle cerebellar peduncle
6 = Sigmoid sinus
7 = Petrous temporal bone and mastoid air cells
8 = Cerebellopontine angle
9 = Pons
10 = Pituitary fossa

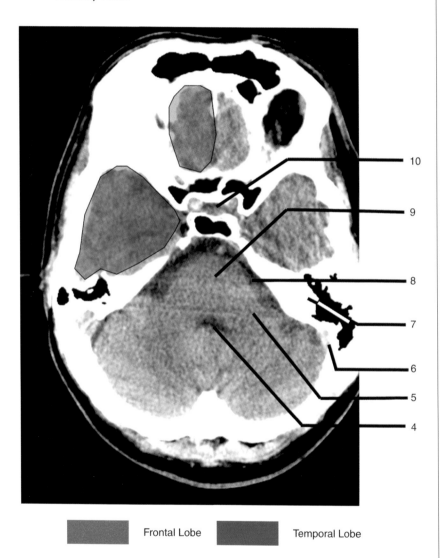

10

9

8

7

6

5

4

Frontal Lobe   Temporal Lobe

11 = Cerebellar vermis
12 = Basilar artery
13 = Prepontine cistern
14 = Dorsum sellae
15 = Temporal horn of lateral ventricle

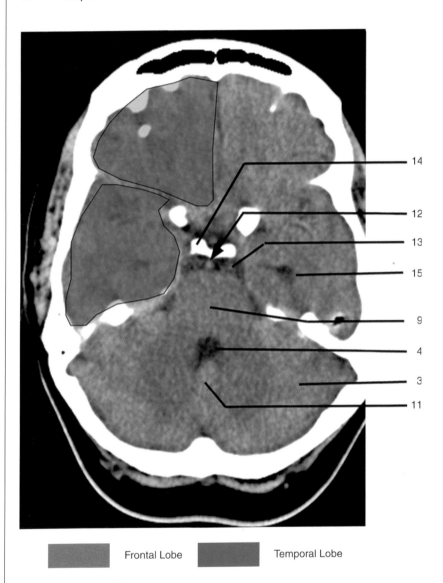

Frontal Lobe   Temporal Lobe

16 = Ambient cistern
17 = Interpeduncular cistern
18 = Cerebral peduncle
19 = Sylvian fissure

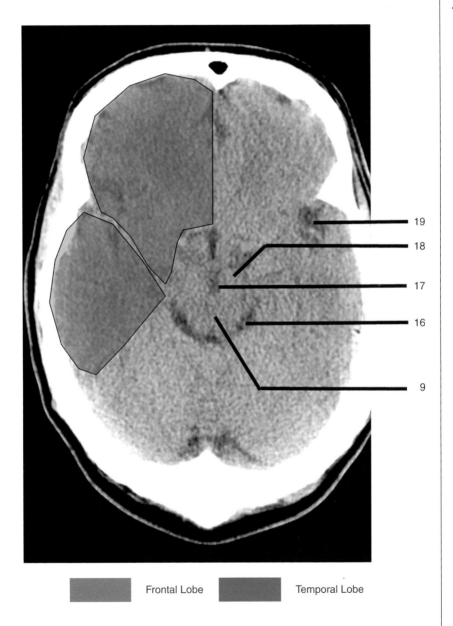

19

18

17

16

9

Frontal Lobe   Temporal Lobe

20 = Supra vermian cistern
21 = Frontal horn of lateral ventricle
21a = Third ventricle

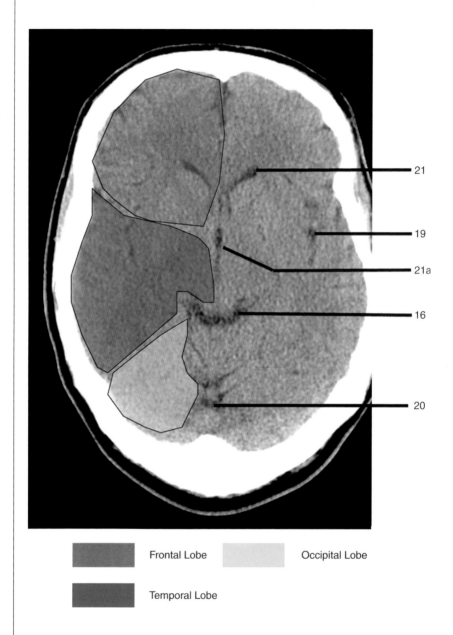

Frontal Lobe		Occipital Lobe
Temporal Lobe		

22 = Head of caudate nucleus
23 = Insular cortex
24 = External capsule
25 = Lentiform nucleus
26 = Thalamus

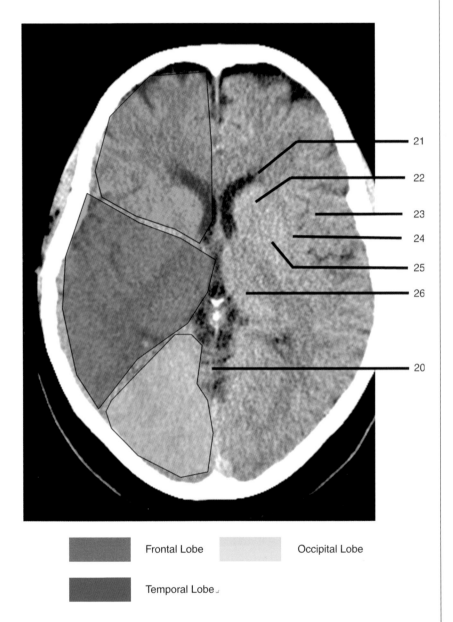

▬ Frontal Lobe	▬ Occipital Lobe	
▬ Temporal Lobe		

27 = Interhemispheric fissure
28 = Anterior limb of internal capsule
29 = Genu of internal capsule
30 = Posterior limb of internal capsule
31 = Trigone of lateral ventricle and calcified choroid plexus
32 = Occipital horn of lateral ventricle

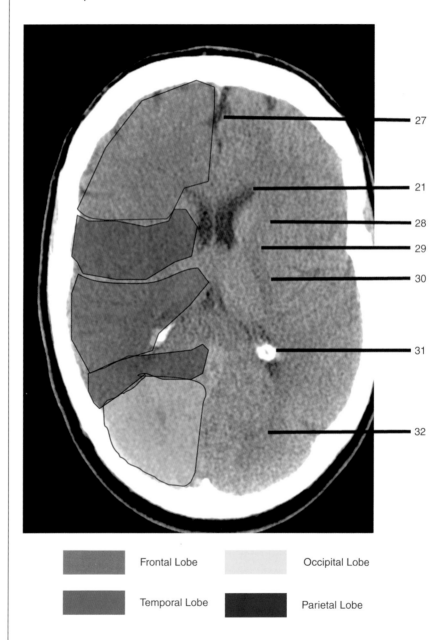

Frontal Lobe   Occipital Lobe

Temporal Lobe   Parietal Lobe

33 = Body of lateral ventricle
34 = Corona radiata

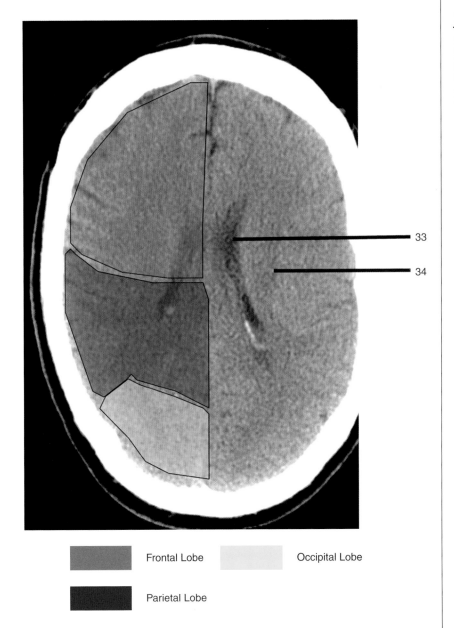

33

34

Frontal Lobe   Occipital Lobe

Parietal Lobe

35 = Centrum semiovale
FB = Frontal bone
PB = Parietal bone
OB = Occipital bone

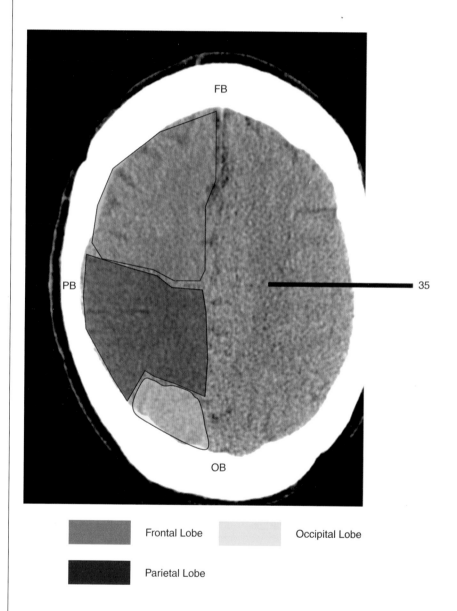

Frontal Lobe   Occipital Lobe

Parietal Lobe

36 = Pre-central gyrus
37 = Central sulcus
38 = Post-central gyrus

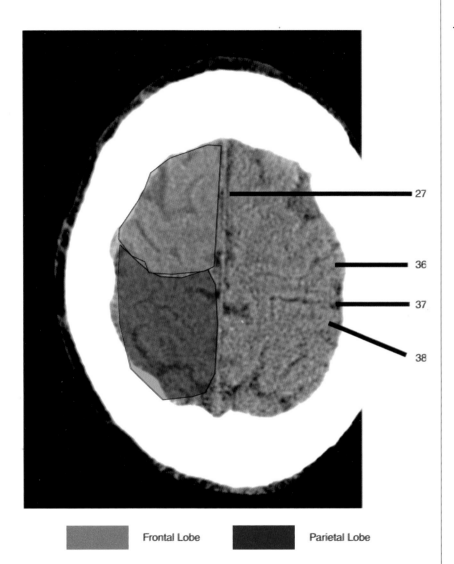

| 27 | 36 | 37 | 38 |

Frontal Lobe   Parietal Lobe

39 = Superior sagittal sinus.

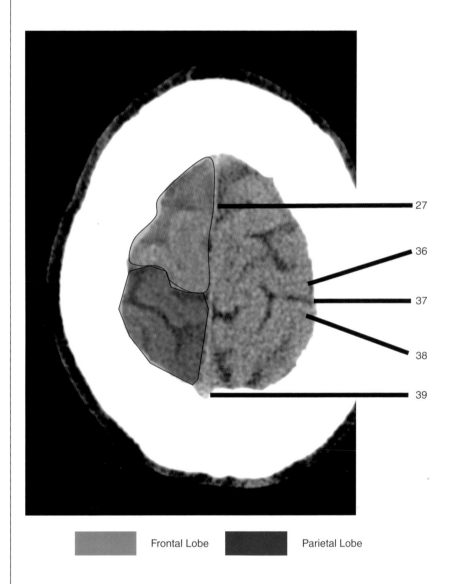

27

36

37

38

39

Frontal Lobe   Parietal Lobe

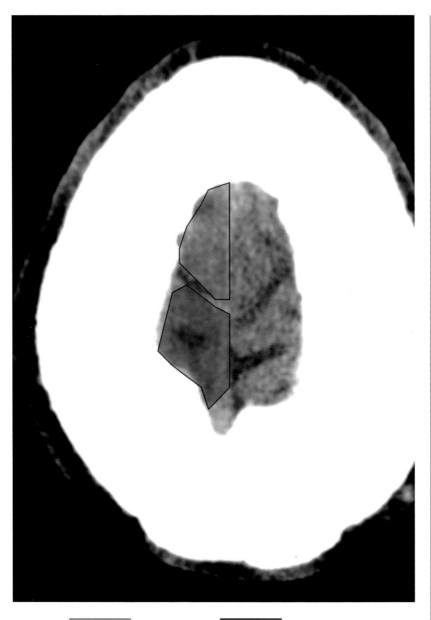

Frontal Lobe   Parietal Lobe

Review of vascular territories

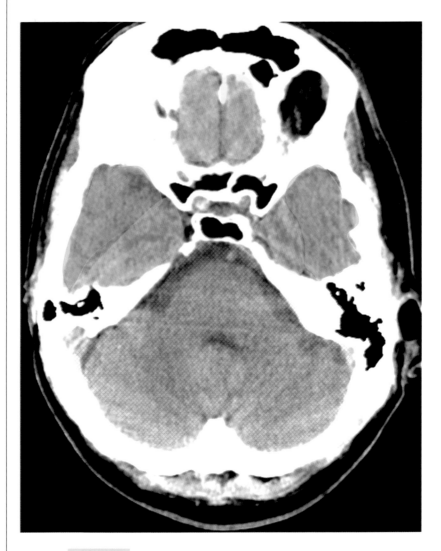

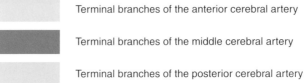

Terminal branches of the anterior cerebral artery

Terminal branches of the middle cerebral artery

Terminal branches of the posterior cerebral artery

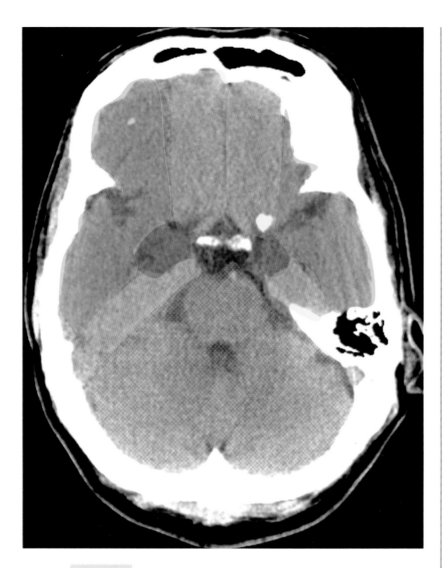

Terminal branches of the anterior cerebral artery

Terminal branches of the middle cerebral artery

Anterior choroidal artery

Terminal branches of the posterior cerebral artery

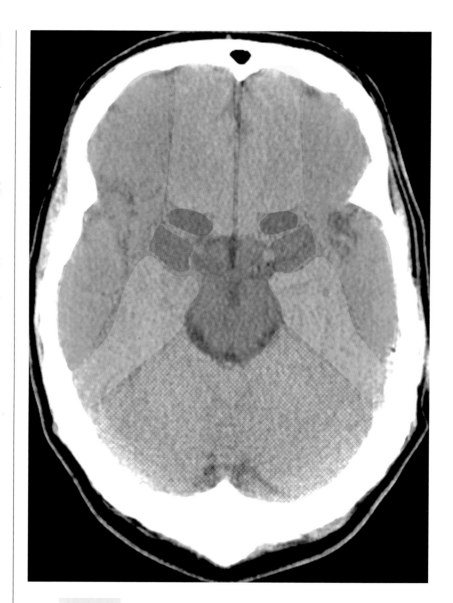

Terminal branches of the anterior cerebral artery

Terminal branches of the middle cerebral artery

Anterior choroidal artery

Terminal branches of the posterior cerebral artery

Penetrating branches of the anterior cerebral artery

Penetrating branches of the posterior cerebral artery and posterior communicating artery

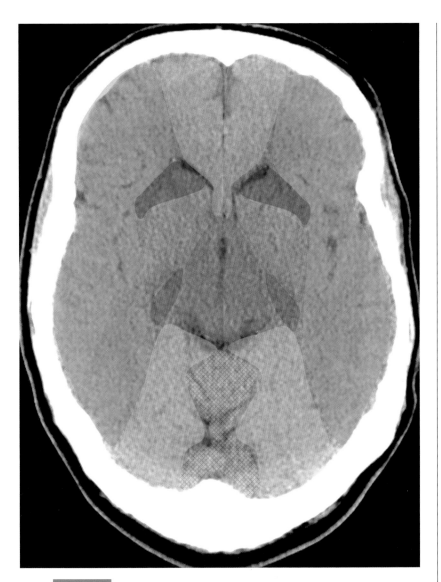

Penetrating branches of the middle cerebral artery

Terminal branches of the anterior cerebral artery

Terminal branches of the middle cerebral artery

Anterior choroidal artery

Terminal branches of the posterior cerebral artery

Penetrating branches of the anterior cerebral artery

Penetrating branches of the posterior cerebral artery and posterior communicating artery

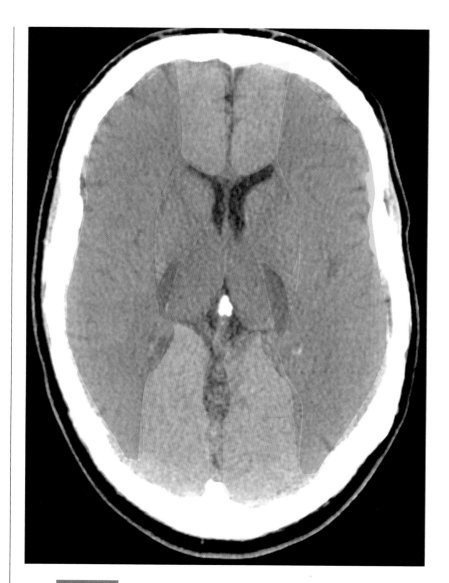

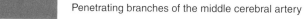 Penetrating branches of the middle cerebral artery

Terminal branches of the anterior cerebral artery

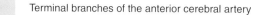 Terminal branches of the middle cerebral artery

Terminal branches of the posterior cerebral artery

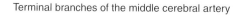 Penetrating branches of the posterior cerebral artery and posterior communicating artery

Anterior choroidal artery

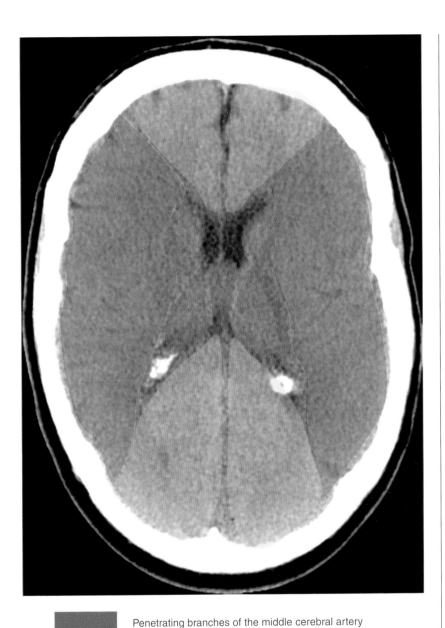

Penetrating branches of the middle cerebral artery

Terminal branches of the anterior cerebral artery

Terminal branches of the middle cerebral artery

Terminal branches of the posterior cerebral artery

Penetrating branches of the posterior cerebral artery and posterior communicating artery

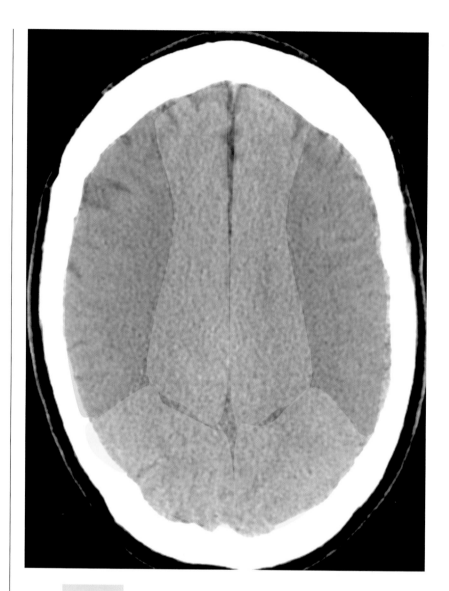

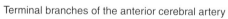 Terminal branches of the anterior cerebral artery

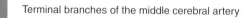 Terminal branches of the middle cerebral artery

Terminal branches of the posterior cerebral artery

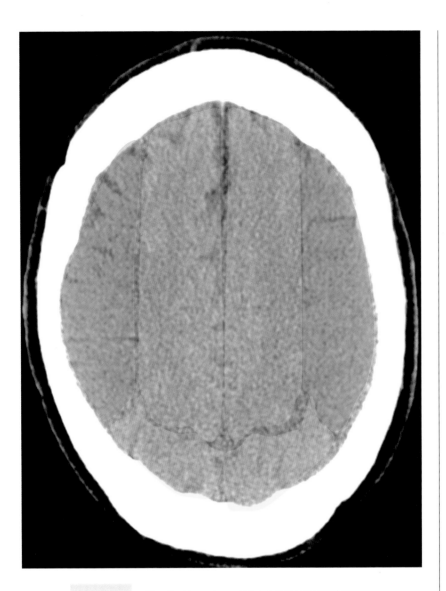

Terminal branches of the anterior cerebral artery

Terminal branches of the middle cerebral artery

Terminal branches of the posterior cerebral artery

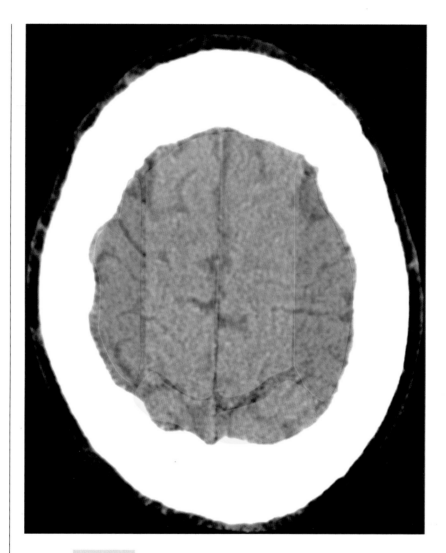

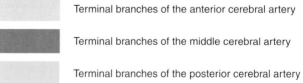

Terminal branches of the anterior cerebral artery

Terminal branches of the middle cerebral artery

Terminal branches of the posterior cerebral artery

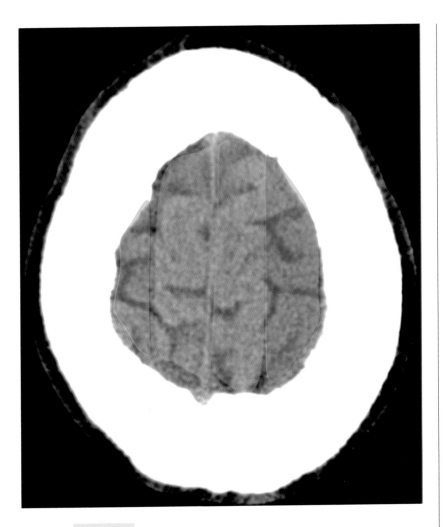

Terminal branches of the anterior cerebral artery

Terminal branches of the middle cerebral artery

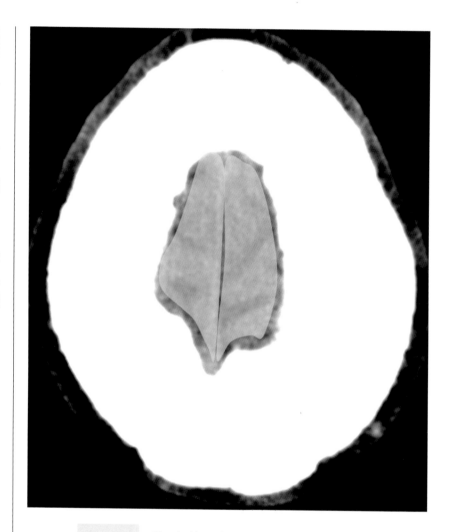

Terminal branches of the anterior cerebral artery

Review of vascular anatomy

Key for vascular anatomy

1 Anterior cerebral artery
2 Middle cerebral artery
3 Internal carotid artery
4 Right vertebral artery
5 Cortical branches of the middle cerebral artery
6 Posterior cerebral artery
7 Basilar artery
8 Left vertebral artery

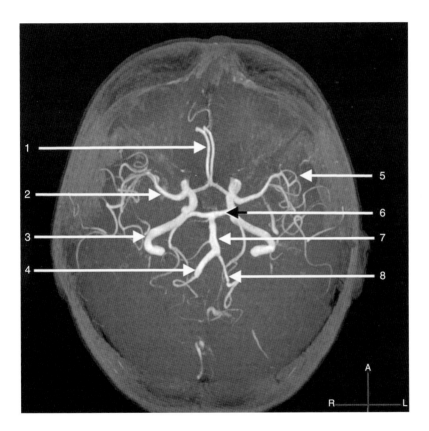

SECTION 2

Reviewing a CT scan

Suggested systematic approach to interpretation

- Check patient information and review scan protocol (e.g. non-contrast/contrast enhanced).
- Check the scout image. May reveal a fracture or gross abnormality not obvious on the axial images. Review alignment of upper cervical vertebrae.
- A quick 'first pass' is recommend, noting gross pathology, followed by a more detailed analysis of the images.
  Use the mnemonic *'ABBCS'* to remember important structures.
- Finally, extend search pattern to include orbits, sinuses, oropharynx, ears, craniocervical junction, face, vault and scalp.

ABBCS

- '**A**' – *Asymmetry* – Assess all slices comparing one side with another, remembering to allow for head tilt and to account for various forms of artefact.
- '**B**' – *Blood* – Acute haemorrhage appears hyperdense in relation to brain, due to clot retraction and water loss. Haemorrhage typically has a CT number in the range of 50–100 HU.
  - Assess for both blood overlying the cerebral hemispheres, and within the brain parenchyma.
  - Assess the ventricles and CSF spaces for the presence or layering of blood.
  - Review the sulci and fissures for subtle evidence of a SAH.
  - Remember slow-flowing blood within a vessel can mimic clot. Conversely clot within a vessel is an important diagnosis:
    - Venous sinus thrombosis
    - Dense MCA sign in acute CVA
- '**B**' – *Brain*
  - **Abnormal density**
    - Hyperdensity – acute blood (free and within vessels), tumour, bone, contrast and artefact/foreign body.
    - Hypodensity – oedema/infarct, air and tumour.
  - **Displacement**
    - Look for midline shift.
    - Examine midline structures such as the falx cerebri, pituitary and pineal glands.
    - Look for asymmetry of CSF spaces such as effacement of an anterior horn of the lateral ventricles or loss of sulcal pattern suggesting oedema.

- Assess for effacement of the basal cisterns and tonsillar herniation at the foramen magnum, as an indicator of raised intracranial pressure.
- **Grey/white matter differentiation**
  - Normal grey/white matter differentiation should be readily apparent; white matter is of slightly reduced attenuation in comparison to grey matter due to increased fatty myelin content.
  - In an early infarct, oedema leads to loss of the normal grey/white matter differentiation. This can be subtle and again only apparent when comparing both sides; identify normal structures such as internal capsule, thalamus, lentiform and caudate nuclei.
- 'C' – *CSF spaces* – Cisterns, sulci and ventricles
  - Assess the sizes of the ventricles and sulci, in proportion to each other and the brain parenchyma.
  - Identify normal cisterns (quadrigeminal plate, suprasellar and the mid brain region) and fissures (interhemispheric and Sylvian).
  - The ventricles often hold the key to analysing the image:
    - Pathology may be primary, within a ventricle, or may result from secondary compression from adjacent brain pathology.
    - If a ventricle is enlarged, consider whether it is due to an obstructive/non-communicating or non-obstructive cause. The former depends on site and the latter usually involves pathology in the subarachnoid space.
    - Dilatation *ex vacuo* is caused by loss/atrophy of brain tissue, often resulting in abnormal secondary enlargement of the adjacent ventricle. Small ventricles can be normal in children (increases in size with age).
    - Diffuse brain swelling can result in ventricular compression and reduced conspicuity of the normal sulcal/gyral pattern. Causes include metabolic/anoxic injury, infection, trauma and superior sagittal sinus thrombosis.
- 'S' – *Skull and scalp* – Assess the scalp for soft tissue injury.
  - Can be useful in patients where a full history is absent.
  - Can help to localise coup and contracoup injuries.
  - Carefully assess the bony vault underlying a soft tissue injury for evidence of a fracture.
  - Assess the bony vault for shape, symmetry and mineralisation (focal sclerotic or lytic lesions).
  - Remember to adjust windowing to optimise bony detail.

Acute stroke

Ischaemic stroke

Characteristics

- Stroke is the third most common cause of death in the UK, and the leading cause of disability.
- 80% of strokes are ischaemic
  - Large vessel occlusive atheromatous disease (50%)
  - Small vessel disease of penetrating arteries (25%) = lacunar infarct
  - Cardiogenic emboli (20%)
  - Non-atheromatous causes (5%)
- Ischaemic infarction of the brain may be secondary to thrombosis or embolic disease.
- Transient ischaemic attacks (TIAs) precede a quarter of ischaemic strokes, and over 40% of these are in the 7 days before the stroke. The risk is highest in those patients with carotid stenosis or artial fibrillation.
- The incidence of stroke increases with age, although one in four people who experience a stroke are under 65 yrs.
- Risk factors include hypertension, smoking, diabetes, hyperlipidaemia, atherosclerosis, atrial fibrillation, the oral contraceptive pill and obesity.

Temporal classification

- TIA = transient ischaemic attack. The clinical syndrome lasts less than 24 hours, although in a proportion there may be infarction on cerebral imaging.
- Progressing stroke = stepwise or gradually progressing accumulative neurological deficit evolving over hours or days
- Completed stroke = persistent stable neurological deficit – cerebral infarction as end stage of prolonged ischemia.
  - Thrombolysis therapy has the potential to revolutionise the rapid assessment and treatment of ischaemic strokes **(see Appendix 2)**

Clinical features

- Spectrum of presentation from mild symptoms and signs, in a well patient, to a moribund comatosed patient.
- Commonly presents with unilateral weakness and/or sensory loss, visual field defect, dysphasia, and inattention/neglect.

- Lacunar infarcts typically present with a purely motor and/or sensory deficit. Features of cortical involvement (visual field defect, dysphasia or inattention/neglect) are absent.
- Posterior circulation infarcts commonly present with vertigo, ataxia, diplopia, dysarthria, dysphasia or bilateral limb signs.
- The neurological deficit can be sudden, often occurring during sleep. This makes the time of onset difficult to ascertain.

Radiological features

CT features

- *Hyperacute infarct (< 12 hours):*
  - Non-contrast CT may appear normal in up to 60%.
  - However, contrary to general opinion, the CT may be abnormal in up to 75% of patients with MCA infarction, imaged within the first 3 hours.
  - 'Hyperdense MCA' sign represents acute intraluminal thrombus, and is seen in 25–50% of acute MCA occlusions. It is recognised as focal or linear white density within the MCA in the Sylvian fissure. Although not sensitive, it is a relatively specific sign.
  - The normally well-defined lentiform nucleus becomes obscured in 50–80% of acute MCA occlusions.
- *Acute infarction*
  - ★ *12–24 hours*
  - Low-density basal ganglia
  - Loss of normal grey/white differentiation secondary to oedema
  - Look for 'the insular ribbon sign' = hypodense extreme capsule no longer distinguishable from insular cortex.
  - Loss of the normal sulcal pattern is suspicious of underlying oedema.
  - ★ *1–7 days*
  - Area of hypodensity in a vascular distribution (in 70%) due to cyto-toxic oedema
  - Mass effect – local or generalised compression of the ventricles, basal cisterns and midline shift.
  - Haemorrhagic transformation may occur after 2–4 days in up to 70%.
- *Subacute/chronic infarction (> 7 days – months)*
  - Decrease of mass effect and *ex vacuo* dilatation of ventricles.
  - Loss of parenchymal mass, with associated sulcal/ventricular widening, due to encephalomalacia.

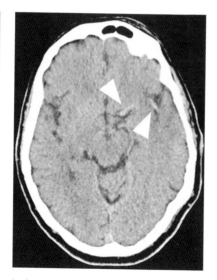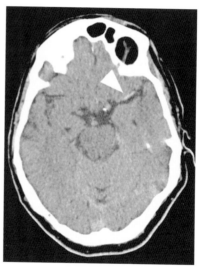

Left MCA territory infarcts: two examples of a hyperdense left MCA due to acute intraluminal thrombus (arrowheads).

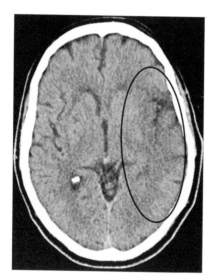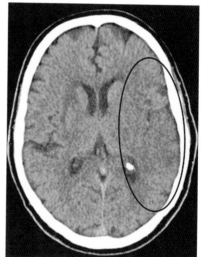

Two examples of early left MCA territory infarction. Note the subtle effacement of grey/white matter differentiation, due to oedema, and the 'insular ribbon sign'.

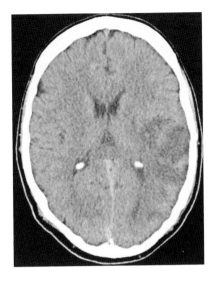
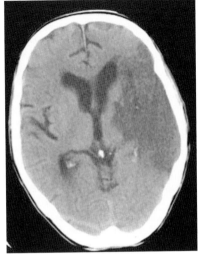
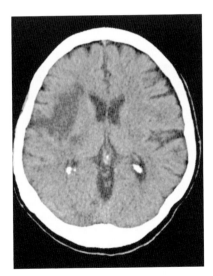
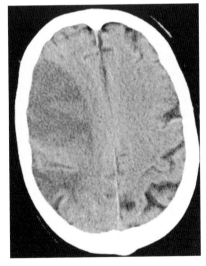

Large areas of hypodensity within the left (top images) and right (bottom images) middle cerebral artery vascular territories, due to cytotoxic oedema.

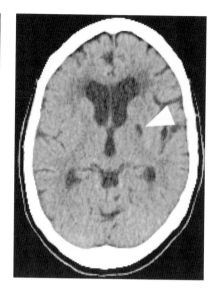

Lacunar infarct left lentiform nucleus (arrowhead).

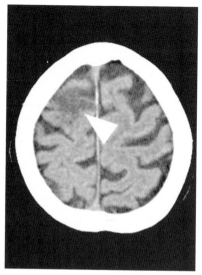

Infarct right superior frontal lobe (arrowhead).

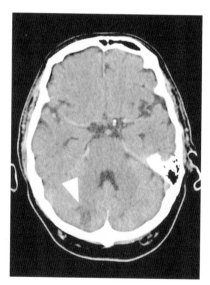

Small cerebellar infarct (arrowhead).

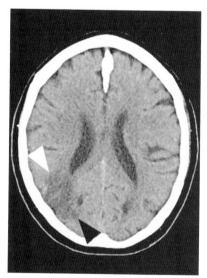

Right posterior watershed infarct. This is an infarct at the 'watershed' between middle and posterior cerebral artery territories (arrowheads).

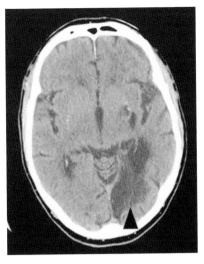

Posterior cerebral artery territory infarct (arrowhead).

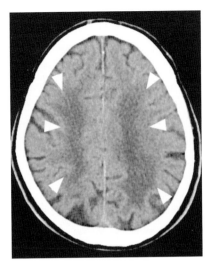

Generalised low attenuation within the deep white matter of both cerebral hemispheres due to small vessel disease (arrowheads).

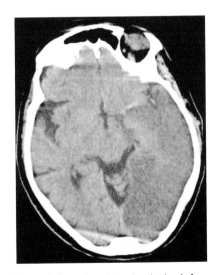

Large infarct involving both the left middle and posterior cerebral artery territories.

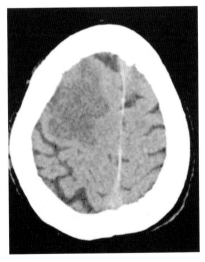

Another example of a right superior frontal lobe infarct.

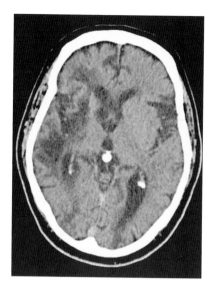 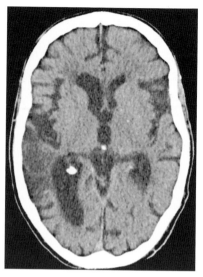

Chronic right MCA territory infarction. The infarcted area is of 'CSF' density due to loss of brain substance, secondary to encephalomalacia, i.e. CSF eventually fills the 'dead' space left following infarction. As a result, there is widening of local sulcal spaces and *ex vacuo* dilatation of adjacent ventricles, in this case the Sylvian fissure and right occipital horn, respectively.

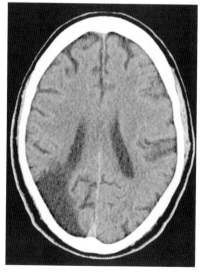 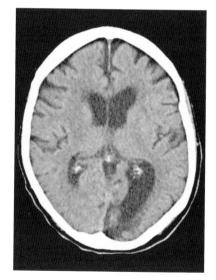

Chronic right posterior watershed infarct.

Chronic left posterior cerebral artery territory infarct with *ex vacuo* dilatation of the left occipital horn.

Haemorrhagic stroke

Characteristics

- Haemorrhagic strokes account for only 10–15% of CVAs.
- Haemorrhagic stroke is associated with a high mortality rate, with only about 40% of patients surviving the first year.
- Small intracerebral arteries, often damaged by chronic hypertension, rupture and blood leaks directly into the parenchyma.
- Haematoma, with resulting oedema, leads to mass effect and further compromise to blood supply.
- In patients who present early, about a third will have haematoma expansion over the first few hours.
- Risk factors:
  - Hypertension, underlying brain pathology, bleeding diatheses, anti-coagulation treatment, thrombolysis therapy and cocaine abuse.

Clinical features

- Haemorrhagic and ischaemic strokes are difficult to distinguish clinically.
- Patients with haemorrhagic strokes are generally sicker, with abrupt onset and rapid deterioration.
- Common symptoms are headache, decreased conscious level, seizures, nausea and vomiting. Hypertension is characteristic.
- ECG changes may include myocardial ischaemia or dysrhythmias.

Radiological features

- Non-contrast head CT is the investigation of choice.
  - Acute haemorrhage is hyperdense.
  - Surrounding oedema will result in loss of the grey/white matter differentiation.
  - Mass effect will result in compression of overlying sulci, ventricular compression, midline shift and reduction in the size of the basal cisterns.
  - Site and size of the haemorrhage are important, and will influence future treatment options.

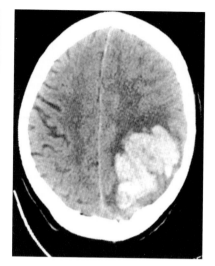

Large acute left parieto-occipital parenchymal haemorrhage.

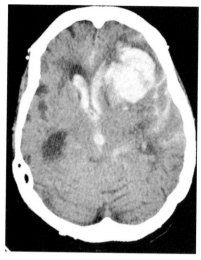

Right frontal haemorrhage with rupture in to the adjacent ventricles and further subarachnoid haemorrhage.

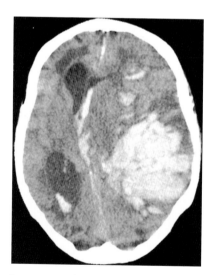

Large acute haemorrhage within the left middle cerebral artery territory, with rupture in to the ventricular system and mass effect.

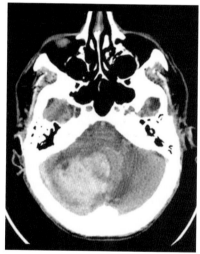

Acute parenchymal haemorrhage within the right cerebellar hemisphere.

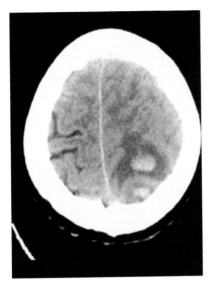

Acute left superior parietal haemorrhage.

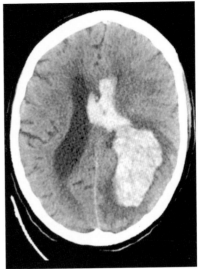

Large acute left parieto-occipital haemorrhage with rupture into the ventricular system.

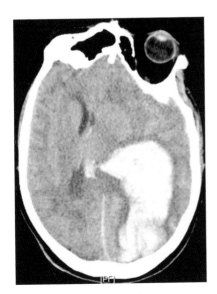

Large acute left occipital haemorrhage with significant associated mass effect.

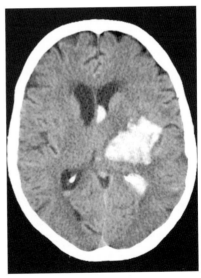

Acute haemorrhage centred on the left thalamus and lentiform nucleus with intraventricular rupture.

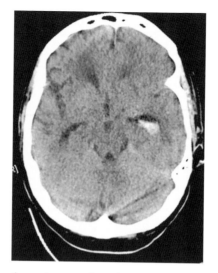

Acute haemorrhage layering in the left temporal horn.

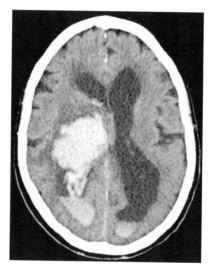

Acute haemorrhage centred on the right thalamus and lentiform nucleus with intraventricular rupture.

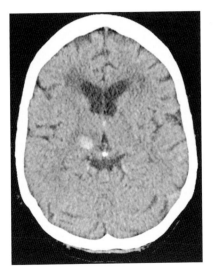

Small acute right thalamic
haemorrhage.

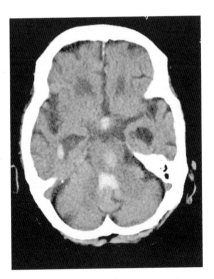

Acute intraventricular haemorrhage.
Additional acute focal haemorrhage
within the central pons.

Subdural haematoma (SDH)

Characteristics

- Subdural haemorrhage arises between the inner layer of dura and arachnoid membrane of the brain.
- Bleeding results from torn bridging veins that cross the potential space between the cerebral cortex and dural venous sinuses.
- May be acute, subacute or chronic. 10% are bilateral.
- Acute SDH carries a high mortality and morbidity. Direct pressure results in ischaemia on the adjacent brain.
- Rebleeding secondary to osmotic expansion, or further trauma, leads to acute on chronic haemorrhage.
- The aetiology of chronic SDH is often unclear. Most likely from minor trauma in the preceding few weeks. In 50% of cases no such history is obtainable.
- Subdural haematomas are more common in elderly and alcoholic patients, where the subdural spaces are larger due to age related involution and/or atrophy.
  - Subdural haemorrhage in the newborn is usually due to obstetric trauma. In neonates, non-accidental injury needs to be considered.

Clinical features

Acute SDH

- Patients often present following severe head trauma.
- Associated with underlying brain injury (50%) with a worse long-term prognosis than extradural haematoma.
- Patients generally have a decreased level of consciousness with focal neurological defects or seizures. There may be signs of raised intracranial pressure.
- Patients with a primary or secondary coagulopathy (e.g. alcoholics) may develop an acute SDH after only minor head trauma.
- A small acute SDH may be asymptomatic.

Chronic SDH

- Chronic SDH is the result of:
  - Resolving phase of medically managed acute subdural haematoma.
  - Repeated episodes of subclinical haemorrhage until becoming symptomatic.
- Chronic SDH often presents in the elderly with vague symptoms of gradual depression, personality changes, fluctuations of consciousness, unexplained headaches or evolving hemiplegia.

- Predisposing factors: alcoholism, increased age, epilepsy, coagulopathy and prior placement of ventricular shunt.
  - Over 75% occur in patients >50 years of age!

Radiological features

- *Location*
  - Blood is seen over the cerebral convexity, often extending into the interhemispheric fissure, along the tentorial margins, and beneath the temporal and occipital lobes.
  - Do *not* cross the midline.
  - Bilateral in 15–25% of adults (common in elderly) and in 80–85% in infants.

CT features

Acute SDH

- Peripheral *high density* crescentic fluid collection between the skull and cerebral hemisphere usually with:
  - A concave inner margin. A small haematoma may only minimally press into brain substance.
  - Convex outer margin following normal contour of cranial vault.
  - Occasionally with a blood–fluid level.
- Signs of mass effect with compression of overlying sulci, ventricular compression, midline shift and reduction in the size of the basal cisterns.

Subacute SDH

- After approximately 1 to 2 weeks the subdural collection becomes *isodense* to grey matter; therefore detection may be challenging and only be recognised due to persistent mass effect:
  - Effacement of cortical sulci.
  - Deviation of lateral ventricle.
  - Midline shift, white matter buckling.
  - Displacement of grey white matter interfaces.
- Contrast enhancement will often define cortical–subdural interface.

Chronic SDH

- After approximately 2 weeks, chronic SDH's are often *hypodense* crescentic collections, with or without mass effect.
- *Acute-on-chronic SDHs* can further complicate the images, with hyperdense fresh haemorrhage intermixed, or layering posteriorly, within the chronic collection.
- Complex septated collections, and in rare cases calcification, may develop.

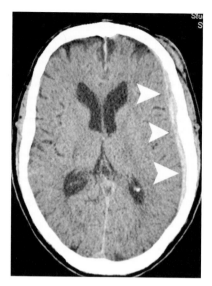

Shallow acute left subdural haematoma (arrows).

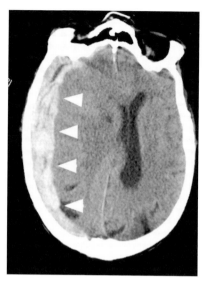

Large acute right subdural haematoma (arrowheads).

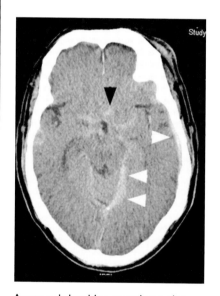

Acute subdural haemorrhage along the tentorium and over the left temporal lobe (white arrowheads). Additional subarachnoid haemorrhage (black arrowhead).

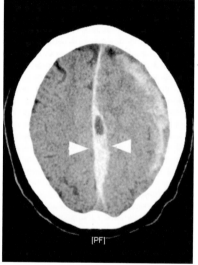

Acute subdural haematoma over the left cerebral convexity, with an additional acute on chronic inter-hemispheric subdural collection (arrowheads).

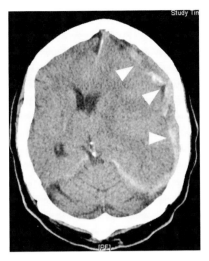

Mixed density left subdural collection (arrowheads) with significant mass effect and midline shift to the right.

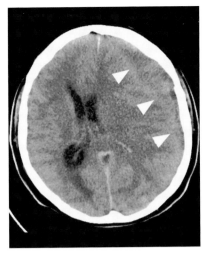

Left isodense/hypodense subdural collection (arrowheads) with midline shift to the right.

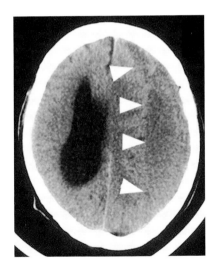

Large left isodense/ hypodense subdural haematoma (arrowheads) with associated mass effect.

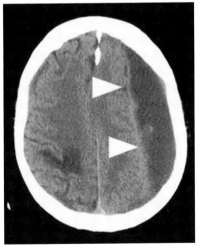

Large left chronic subdural haematoma (arrowheads).

Extradural haematoma

Characteristics

- An extradural haemorrhage arises within the potential space between the skull and dura.
- The young are more frequently affected as the dura is more easily stripped away from the skull. The dura becomes more adherent with age.
- 2% of all serious head injuries. Less than 1% of all children with cranial trauma. Rarely, extradural haematomas can occur spontaneously.
- Associated with a skull fracture in 75–95% of cases.
- Most commonly bleeding is from a lacerated (middle) meningeal artery/vein, adjacent to the inner table, from a fracture of the adjacent calvarium.
- Early diagnosis is imperative, as prognosis is good with early intervention. Conversely, a delay may result in cerebral herniation and brainstem compression.
- *Types*
  - Acute extradural haematoma (60%) from arterial bleeding.
  - Subacute haematoma (30%).
  - Chronic haematoma (10%) from venous bleeding.

Clinical features

- Patients often present with a history of head trauma.
- Associated with a variable level of consciousness. 20% to 50% have a brief loss of consciousness at the time of impact. As the haematoma continues to expand, they suffer a rapid deterioration. This lucid interval is referred to as the 'talk and die' presentation.
- Neurological examination may reveal lateralising signs with a unilateral up-going plantar response.
- A sensitive sign in the conscious patient is pronator drift of the upper limb, when asked to hold both arms outstretched with the palms upwards.
- Close neurological observation is necessary to detect rising intracranial pressure; clinically, an escalating blood pressure with associated bradycardia.

Radiological features

- *Location*
  - 66% temporoparietal (most often from laceration of middle meningeal artery).

- 29% frontal pole, parieto-occipital region, between occipital lobes and posterior fossa (most often from laceration of the dural sinuses from a fracture).
- Disruption of the sagittal sinus may create a vertex epidural haematoma.

CT features

- Biconvex hyperdense elliptical collection with a sharply defined edge.
- Mixed density suggests active bleeding.
- Haematoma does *not* cross suture lines unless a diastatic suture fracture is present.
- May separate the venous sinuses and falx from the skull; this is the only type of intracranial haemorrhage to do this.
- Mass effect depends on the size of the haemorrhage and associated oedema.
- Venous bleeding is more variable in shape.
- Associated fracture line may be seen.

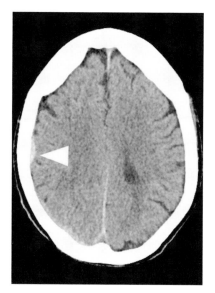

Subtle acute extradural haemorrhage
(arrow).

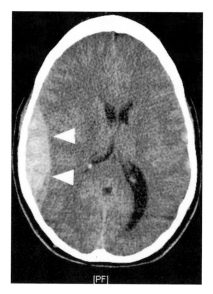

Acute right extradural haemorrhage
(arrowheads).

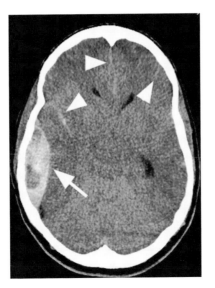

Right extradural haemorrhage.
The collection (arrow) is hyperdense
and isodense indicating both acute and
subacute haemorrhage. In addition,
there is evidence of subarachnoid
haemorrhage (arrowheads).

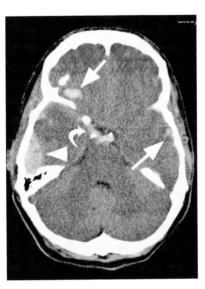

Acute extradural haemorrhage
(arrowhead), subarachnoid
haemorrhage (curved arrow) and
multifocal contusions (arrows).

Subarachnoid haemorrhage

Characteristics

- Subarachnoid haemorrhage accounts for 10% of CVAs.
- *Causes*
  - Spontaneous – ruptured aneurysm (72%), AVM (10%) and hypertensive haemorrhage.
  - Trauma.
- Blood enters the subarachnoid space onto the surface of the brain, between the pia and arachnoid, and may lead to raised intracranial pressure by obstructing the ventricular outflow of CSF.
- Incidence increases with age and peaks at age 50 years. Approximately 80% of cases of SAH occur in people aged 40–65 years, with 15% occurring in people aged 20–40 years.
- 40–50% of patients with aneurysmal SAH have symptoms from a 'sentinel' bleed, 10–20 days prior to rupture.
- Morbidity can be severe and is increased by rebleeding, which often occurs in the first few days, and cerebral vasospasm 7 to 14 days after the initial event. 45% mortality within 8 weeks.
- Berry aneurysms are associated with hypertension, polycystic kidney disease, SLE, connective tissue disorders, AVMs and long term analgesic use.
- In 20% of non-traumatic SAH's, no lesion is found at post-mortem.

Clinical features

- SAH classically presents with a sudden onset of a severe 'thunderclap' occipital headache, often described as the 'worst headache in their life'.
- Associated with physical or emotional stress, coitus or head trauma.
- 30–40% occur at rest.
- A leading cause of maternal mortality, accounting for 6–25% of maternal deaths during pregnancy.
- Meningeal irritation generates symptoms of neck stiffness, photophobia and low back pain, with a positive Kernig's sign.
- Focal neurological signs include third nerve palsy from compression by an expanding berry aneurysm of the posterior communicating artery of the Circle of Willis.
- Consider SAH in the comatosed or fitting patient.
- Fundoscopy may reveal papilloedema and subhyaloid retinal haemorrhages.
- Lumbar puncture (LP) is performed 12 hours after the onset of symptoms to evaluate xanthochromia. 15% of LPs are falsely negative.

Radiological features

Location of aneurysm rupture

Approximately 85% of saccular aneurysms occur in the anterior circulation. The most common sites of rupture are as follows:
- The internal carotid artery, including the posterior communicating (PCom) junction (41%).
- The anterior communicating (ACom) artery/anterior cerebral artery (34%).
- The middle cerebral artery (MCA) (20%).
- The vertebrobasilar and other arteries (5%).

CT features

- *CT scan without contrast.*
- CT scan findings are positive in approximately 92% of patients who have SAH.
- Sensitivity decreases with time from onset of ictus.
  - ≈ 98% within the first 12 hours and 93% within 24 hours.
  - Decreases to ≈ 80% at 72 hours and 50% at 1 week.
  - May be falsely negative in patients with small hemorrhages and in those with severe anaemia.
- The location of blood within the subarachnoid space correlates directly with the location of the aneurysm rupture in 70% of cases.
  - Blood localised to the basal cisterns, the Sylvian or intrahemispheric fissures suggests rupture of a saccular aneurysm.
  - Blood found lying over the cerebral convexities or within the superficial brain parenchyma suggests rupture of an AVM or mycotic aneurysm.
- ACom artery aneurysms are often associated with interhemispheric and intraventricular haemorrhages.
- MCA and PCom artery aneurysms are associated with intraparenchymal haemorrhages.
- Serial CT allows for surveillance of developing mass effect and hydrocephalus; up to 20% of patients develop some degree of obstructive hydrocephalus in the first 2 weeks post-ictus.
- *A contrast-enhanced CT scan* may reveal an underlying AVM; however, a non–contrast study should always be performed before considering a contrast study, so as not to interfere with the visualisation of subarachnoid blood.

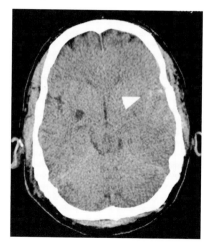 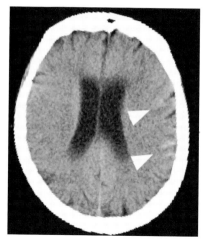

Two examples of subtle subarachnoid haemorrhage. Faint hyperdense subarachnoid blood is seen outlining cerebral sulci (arrowheads).

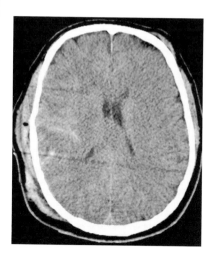 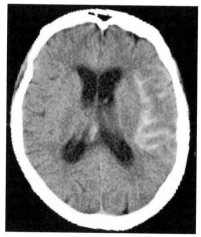

Subarachnoid blood seen predominantly within the right cerebral hemisphere with overlying soft tissue contusion.

Hyperdense subarachnoid blood outlining several sulci within the left cerebral hemisphere.

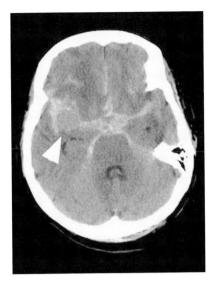 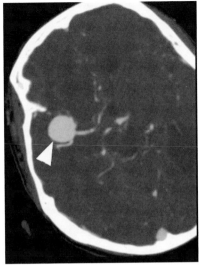

Unenhanced scan and a CT angiogram. Extensive subarachnoid haemorrhage secondary to a ruptured MCA aneurysm (arrowheads).

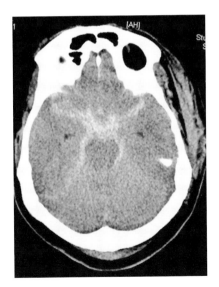 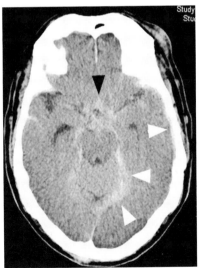

Extensive hyperdense subarachnoid haemorrhage outlining the basal cisterns.

Subarachnoid blood within the suprasellar cistern (black arrowhead). Additional acute subdural haemorrhage along the tentorium and over the left temporal lobe (white arrowheads).

Cerebral venous sinus thrombosis

Characteristics

- Rare cause of stroke, affecting both sexes equally.
- *Risk factors*
  - Septic causes (esp. in childhood):
    - mastoiditis, facial cellulitis, meningitis, encephalitis, brain abscess, intracranial empyema.
  - Aseptic causes:
    - Hypercoagulable states:
      - polycythemia rubra vera, idiopathic thrombocytosis, thrombocytopaenia, pregnancy, oral contraceptive pill.
    - Low-flow state:
      - CCF, shock.
  - In one-third of patients no aetiology is found.

Clinical features

- Classically presents with sudden, severe headache, worsened by coughing and associated with vomiting.
- Focal neurological deficit may be seen if venous infarction occurs. Cranial nerve palsies are characteristic.
- Seizures may occur.
- Sigmoid sinus thrombosis causes cerebellar signs and lower cranial nerve palsies.
- Periorbital oedema and chemosis are seen with cavernous sinus thrombosis.
- Fundoscopy may show papilloedema or retinal vein thrombosis.

Radiological features

CT features

- CT may be normal.
- *Non-contrast CT*
  - Hyperdense material within a vessel representing thrombosed blood. Not reliable as also seen with slow flowing blood.
  - Cerebral infarction not characteristic of an arterial territory.
- *Contrast CT*
  - Look for the 'delta'/'empty triangle' sign (seen in $\approx 70\%$). This is a filling defect within the straight/superior sagittal sinus, and represents flow around a central non-enhanced clot.
  - Gyral enhancement peripheral to an infarct, in 30–40%.
- Co-existing signs of infection or inflammation (e.g. sinusitis/mastoiditis) should raise suspicion.

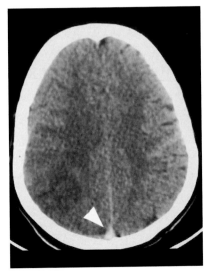 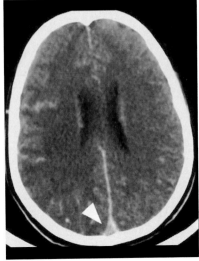

Sagittal sinus thrombosis. Scans pre- and post-contrast. On the pre-contrast study, hyperdense material is seen within the sagittal sinus. This is an unreliable sign for acute thrombus. However, following contrast, the 'delta' sign is clearly visible.

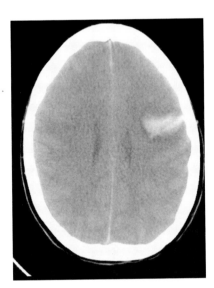 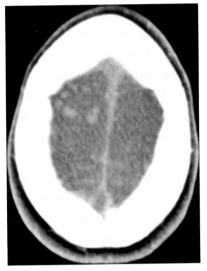

Venous haemorrhage in the left frontoparietal cortex due to sagittal sinus thrombosis.

Image from a CTV demonstrating a filling defect in the SSS anteriorly and posteriorly, representing thrombus. The foci of haemorrhage in the right frontal parenchyma are typical of those seen with sinus thrombosis.

Contusions

Characteristics

- Traumatic injury to cortical surface of brain.
- Commonest form of traumatic cerebral injury:
  - 20% of head injuries.
  - Children:adults = 2:1.
- Usually the result of linear acceleration/deceleration forces or penetrating injuries.
- Often described as 'coup'/'contra-coup' injuries:
  - Coup injury – site of the direct impact on the stationary brain.
  - Contra-coup – site of impact of the moving brain upon the stationary. inner table, opposite to the site of the coup injury.
- Cerebral contusions are also produced secondary to depressed skull fractures and are associated with other intracranial injuries.

Clinical features

- Patients often present with a history of head trauma or external signs of injury.
- Usually associated with a brief loss of consciousness.
- Confusion and altered GCS may be prolonged.
- Headache with vomiting in the conscious patient.
- Focal neurological deficit may occur if contusions arise near the sensorimotor cortex.
- Most patients make an uneventful recovery, but a few develop raised intracranial pressure, post-traumatic seizures and persisting focal neurological deficits.
- Beware the elderly, alcoholics and those taking anticoagulants that are at increased risk of haemorrhage.

Radiological features

CT features

- *Location*
  - Often multiple bilateral lesions at the interface between grey and white matter.
  - Commonly along anterior, lateral and inferior surfaces of frontal and temporal lobes.
  - Less frequently seen in parietal and occipital lobes and the posterior fossa.
- CT sensitive for haemorrhage in the acute post-traumatic period.
- The site of scalp swelling often indicates the site of the coup injury.

- Focal/multiple areas of low attenuation, representing oedema, are intermixed with tiny areas of increased density, representing petechial haemorrhage.
- In children, a common appearance is of diffuse cerebral swelling without haemorrhage in the acute post-traumatic period.
- True extent becomes apparent over time with progression of cell necrosis, oedema and mass effect.

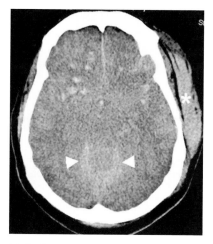

Multi-focal contusions within both frontal lobes, with additional acute subarachnoid haemorrhage on the tentorium (arrowheads). Marked left fronto-parietal soft tissue swelling (astrerisk).

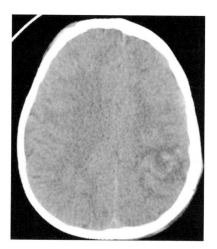

Subtle left parieto-occipital contusions.

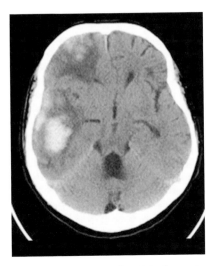

Large contusions in the right frontal and temporal lobes.

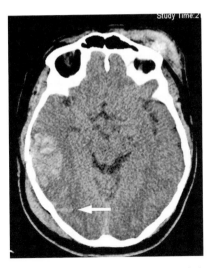

Right temporal contusions, with subtle high density subarachnoid blood outlining sulci posteriorly (arrow). Note the adjacent subcutaneous soft tissue and left frontal swelling.

Skull fractures

Characteristics

- Result from trauma to the head.
- Classified as *linear, depressed* or *base of skull* fractures.
- *Linear fractures* are often uncomplicated and do not require treatment. However temporal bone fractures may result in an extradural haematoma.
- *Depressed skull fractures* may require surgery to elevate the bone fragments to prevent brain injury.
- Increased significance if the fracture is open, or communicates with an adjacent sinus, due to increased risk of infection.
- In *basal skull fractures* prophylactic antibiotics were once routinely prescribed to reduce the risk of meningitis, but their effectiveness is not validated and use is now restricted.

Clinical features

- Open fractures underlie scalp lacerations and are often diagnosed during evaluation of the wound for closure.
- Depressed skull fractures are often palpable or visible during examination but may be masked by swelling around the area.
- Clinical signs of base of skull fracture:
  - CSF rhinorrhoea.
  - Haemotympanum.
  - Bleeding from the external auditory meatus.
  - 'Racoon' eyes.
  - Subconjunctival haemorrhage (with no posterior limit).
  - Battle's sign (bruising over the mastoid area).
  - Cranial nerve deficits.
- Blotting paper may be helpful in diagnosing CSF rhinorrhoea.

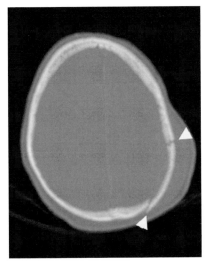

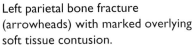

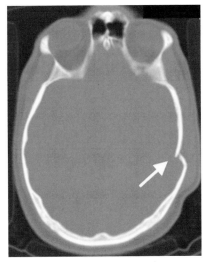

Left parietal bone fracture (arrowheads) with marked overlying soft tissue contusion.

Depressed skull fracture (arrow).

Radiological features

CT features

- Look closely at the initial scout image as this may demonstrate a fracture.
- Soft tissue swelling, or an underlying brain abnormality, may be associated with a fracture.
- Fractures may be missed if appropriate 'window' parameters are not chosen. *Always assess for fractures on bony windows.*
- Fractures appear as sharply defined lines and should not be mistaken for a suture or vascular groove; a vascular groove often branches and both have typical sites.
- The presence of intracranial air may be secondary to an open fracture or connection with an air-containing sinus.

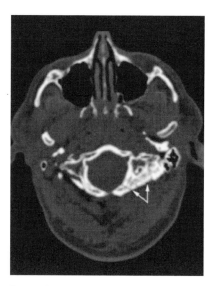

Base of skull fracture (arrows).

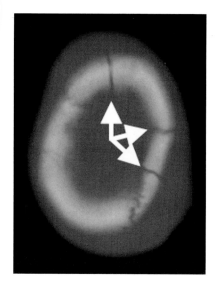

Complex vault fracture (arrows).

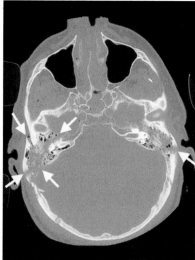

Bilateral comminuted temporal bone fractures (arrows).

Meningitis

Characteristics

- Defined as inflammation of the meninges. Anatomically divided into:
  - Inflammation of the dura, sometimes referred to as pachymeningitis – less common.
  - Inflammation of the arachnoid membrane and subarachnoid space, referred to as leptomeningitis – more common.
- Meningoencephalitis also involves the parenchyma.
- Since the introduction of the haemophilus influenza vaccine, the average age of presentation has risen from 15 months to 25 years.
- Overcrowded closed communities (e.g. schools, day centres) predispose patients to meningitis, especially if immunocompromised. Concurrent illnesses such as pneumonia or other sites of sepsis (e.g. sinusitis, mastoiditis, otitis media) may contribute.
- Despite medical advances morbidity rates remain high.

Clinical features

- Fever, neck stiffness, photophobia, unremitting headache, mental status changes, with CSF findings, are essentials for diagnosis.
- Kernig's sign – pain and resistance on passive knee extension with hips fully flexed.
- Brudzinski's sign – hips flex on bending head forward.
- Seizures and cranial nerve palsies are common.
- Patients may present with signs of raised intracranial pressure.
- Detection at the extremes of age is difficult:
  - Children may present with poor feeding, irritability, lethargy and vomiting.
  - The elderly may only have a low grade fever and delirium.
- CSF sampling reveals raised WCC, predominantly neutrophils, with low glucose and high protein, in cases of bacterial meningitis.

Radiological features

CT features

- *Non-contrast CT* is often normal.
- *Contrast enhanced CT*
  - Enhancement of the meningeal surfaces is a non-specific and often an inconsistent finding in patients with meningitis.
  - When present, enhancement is usually seen over the cerebral convexities and in the interhemispheric and Sylvian fissures.
  - Intense contrast enhancement, with associated meningeal thickening, is suggestive of granulomatous meningitis (such as TB and sarcoidosis).
    - Associated obliteration of the basal cisterns, Sylvian fissures and suprasellar cistern.
- The cerebral sulci may be effaced, with associated flattening of the ventricles, due to cerebral oedema.
- Cerebral infarction is not uncommon.

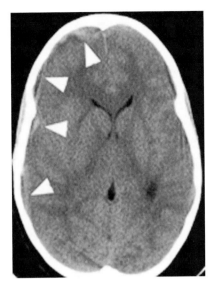

Leptomeningitis: dense haemorrhagic leptomeningeal collection over the right cerebral hemisphere (arrowheads), in a young patient with sinusitis.

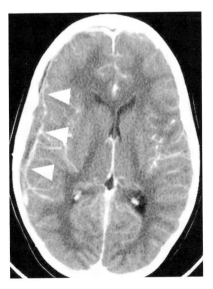

Meningeal enhancement in a patient with pneumococcal meningitis, outlining a subdural empyema (arrowheads).

Raised intracranial pressure

Characteristics

- The skull defines a fixed volume. Increasing the volume of contents, or brain swelling from any cause, rapidly increases intracranial pressure.
- Causes of raised intracranial pressure include:
  - Haemorrhage (subdural, extradural, subarachnoid, intracerebral, intraventricular).
  - Brain abscess.
  - Meningoencephalitis.
  - Primary or metastatic tumours.
  - Hydrocephalus.
  - Cerebral oedema (vasogenic, cytotoxic or interstitial).

Clinical features

- Patients often present with a vague history of listlessness, irritability, drowsiness, early morning headaches, nausea and vomiting.
- The presentation may be acute with sudden neurological deterioration.
- Classic progression of symptoms:
  - Bradycardia.
  - Rising blood pressure.
  - Respiratory depression (Cushings response).
  - Pupillary constriction and then dilation.
- Third nerve palsy – dilated ipsilateral pupil and ophthalmoplegia develop as intracranial pressure increases.
- Papilloedema is an unreliable sign. Look for absence of venous pulsation.

Radiological features

CT features

- CSF spaces are reduced in size with effacement of sulci and the basal cisterns.
- Herniation of brain parenchyma (representing shift of the normal brain, through or across regions, to another site due to mass effect) occurs late.
- Types of cerebral herniation:
  - Subfalcine herniation – most common form of herniation and occurs as the brain extends under the falx in the supratentorial cerebrum.
  - Transtentorial herniation occurs when the brain traverses across the tentorium at the level of the tentorial incisura. Can be divided into *ascending* and *descending* transtentorial herniation.
    - Descending transtentorial herniation is caused by mass effect in the cerebrum which pushes the supratentorial brain through the incisura into the posterior fossa.
    - Ascending transtentorial herniation is caused by mass effect in the posterior fossa which pushes the infratentorial brain through the incisura in an upward direction.
  - Cerebellar tonsillar herniation – cerebellar tonsils are forced through the foramen magnum.

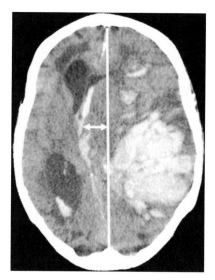

Subfalcine herniation: large left parenchymal haemorrhage with significant associated mass effect. There is midline shift to the right with sub-falcine herniation (arrowheads).

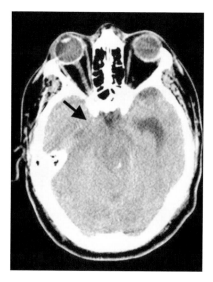

Transtentorial herniation: supratentorial mass effect (cause not shown) pushes the supratentorial brain through the incisura (arrow) into the posterior fossa.

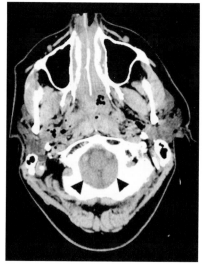

Tonsillar herniation: the cerebellar tonsils descend with increasing intracranial pressure, resulting in crowding of the foramen magnum (arrowheads).

Hydrocephalus

Characteristics

- Hydrocephalus results from an excess of CSF, due to an imbalance between CSF production and absorption, resulting in increased intraventricular pressure.
- Classified as *communicating* and *non-communicating* hydrocephalus:
  - *Communicating hydrocephalus* = elevated intraventricular pressure secondary to obstruction of CSF flow beyond the outlet of 4th ventricle. This may be due to impeded CSF flow over the cerebral convexities and/or impeded reabsorption of CSF by the arachnoid villi.
  - *Causes*
  - Subarachnoid haemorrhage, meningeal metastases and granulomatous meningitis.
  - A less common cause of communicating hydrocephalus results from rapid CSF production, e.g. choroid plexus papilloma.
  - *Non-communicating hydrocephalus* = blockage of CSF flow within the ventricular system, with dilatation proximal to the obstruction.
  - Often referred to as *obstructive hydrocephalus*.
  - *Location of obstruction / causes*:
  - Lateral ventricles, e.g. ependymoma, meningioma.
  - Foramen of Monro, e.g. third ventricular colloid cyst.
  - Third ventricle, e.g. large pituitary adenoma, craniopharyngioma.
  - Aqueduct of Sylvius, e.g. congenital aqueduct stenosis, post intraventricular haemorrhage.
  - Fourth ventricle/foraminae of Luschka and Magendie, e.g. congenital obstruction, intraventricular tumour, extrinsic compression.

Clinical features

- Neonates/infancy. Enlarged cranium, bulging fontanelles, widely separated cranial sutures, vomiting, sleepiness and irritability.
- Older children and adults: headaches, nausea, vomiting, papilloedema, diplopia, problems with balance and coordination, gait disturbance, urinary incontinence, and changes in cognition including memory loss.

Radiological features

- *Non-communicating hydrocephalus*
  - Ventricular dilatation proximal to the level of an obstructing lesion.
    - Dilatation of the occipital horns precedes dilatation of the frontal horns.
    - Commensurate dilatation of the temporal horns with lateral ventricles.

- Progressive enlargement of the ventricular system, disproportionate to narrowed and effaced cortical sulci.
- Periventricular low attenuation is seen with acute onset of hydrocephalus; this represents interstitial oedema from transependymal flow of CSF.
- The obstructing lesion may be evident.
- *Communicating hydrocephalus*
- Symmetrical enlargement of the lateral, third, and fourth ventricles.
- Normal/effaced cerebral sulci.
- Dilatation of subarachnoid cisterns.
- Periventricular low attenuation, secondary to transependymal CSF flow, may be seen with acute onset hydrocephalus.

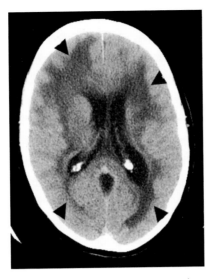

Acute hydrocephalus: periventricular low attenuation is seen (arrows) representing interstitial oedema from transependymal flow of CSF.

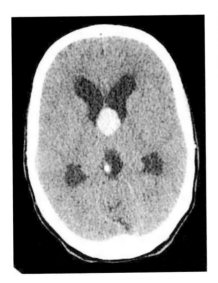

Obstructive hydrocephalus secondary to a hyperdense colloid cyst, at the level of the foramen of Munro. There is resultant dilatation of both frontal horns and trigones, and generalised effacement of cerebral sulci, due to 'brain swelling'.

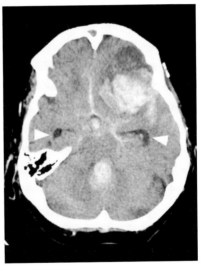

Acute parenchymal, subarachnoid and intraventricular haemorrhage, with resultant dilatation of the temporal horns (arrows) due to developing communicating hydrocephalus.

Abscesses

Characteristics

- Localised purulent bacterial infection often developing in an area of cerebritis.
- *Causes*
  - Extension from adjacent sinonasal infection, mastoiditis, otitis media.
  - Generalised septicaemia:
    - Respiratory causes: bronchiectasis, lung abscesses, empyema and pneumonia.
    - Cardiac causes: right to left shunt, AVM and endocarditis.
    - Osteomyelitis.
  - Penetrating trauma or surgery.
- *Predisposing factors*
  - Diabetes mellitus.
  - Steroids/immunosuppressive therapy.
  - Immune deficiency.
- *Causative organisms*
  - Anaerobic streptococcus (most common).
  - Staphylococcus.
  - Bacteroides.
    - Multiple organisms in 20%.
    - Mycobacterium/salmonella more commonly in developing countries.
  - Toxoplasmosis in AIDS patients.

Clinical features

- Patients may present with headaches, vomiting, seizures, and altered mental state, in association with spiking pyrexia.
- Cranial nerve palsies or localised peripheral neurological deficits may be present.
- Signs of raised intracranial pressure.
- Source of sepsis may be clearly identifiable, or the patient may present with pyrexia of unknown origin.
- Diagnosis and treatment is difficult in those who are immunosuppressed.
- Significant long-term morbidity.
- Complications include cavernous sinus thrombosis, venous infarction and coning.

Radiological features

CT features

- *Location*
  - Supratentorial: infratentorial = 2:1

- Typically at the corticomedullary junction in the frontal and temporal lobes.
- *Non-contrast CT*
  - Low density lesion with associated mass effect.
  - Gas within lesion due to gas-forming organisms.
- *Contrast-enhanced CT*
  - Ring enhancement, with central necrosis, and surrounding oedema.
  - Homogeneous enhancement in lesions < 5 mm.
  - Lesions may be multi-loculated and adjacent daughter abscesses may develop.

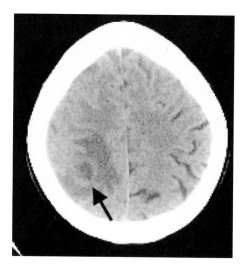

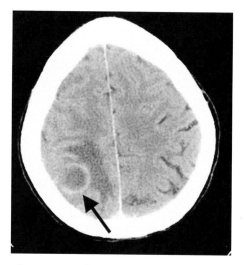

Cerebral abscess. Scan pre- and post-contrast. Right superior parietal ring enhancing lesion (arrows), with surrounding vasogenic oedema.

Arteriovenous malformation

Characteristics

- Congenital abnormality consisting of abnormally dilated tortuous arteries and veins, with closely packed abnormal pathological vessels which shunt blood between the two.
- Most common intracerebral vascular lesion.
- 80% occur by the age of 40; 20% present under 20 years of age.
- May be part of a congenital syndrome, e.g. Sturge–Weber.
- Venous malformations are less common, e.g. medullary venous malformation, cavernous malformation.
- Arterio-venous fistulae are usually post-traumatic.

Clinical features

- Often asymptomatic. 10% are diagnosed incidentally.
- May present with headaches, seizures (non focal in 40%), acute intracranial haemorrhage (50%) or progressive neurological deficit (50%).

Radiological features

Location

- Supratentorial (90%): parietal > frontal > temporal > occipital lobe.
- Infratentorial (10%).

Vascular supply

- Pial branches of ICA in 75% of supratentorial lesions, in 50% of posterior fossa lesions.
- Dural branches of ECA in 25% with infratentorial lesions.

CT features

- *Non-contrast CT*
  - Irregular lesion with large feeding arteries and draining veins.
  - Mixed density lesion (60%), composed of large dense vessels, haemorrhage and calcification.
  - Isodense lesion (15%), which may only be recognisable by associated mass effect.
  - Low-density lesion (15%) due to atrophy secondary to associated local cerebral ischaemia.
  - 10% are not visualised on unenhanced CT.

- *Contrast-enhanced CT*
  - Dense serpiginous enhancement in 80%, representing tortuous dilated vessels.
  - Lack of mass effect and oedema unless thrombosed or secondary haemorrhage.
  - No enhancement in thrombosed AVM.
  - Adjacent brain atrophy due to local cerebral ischaemia.

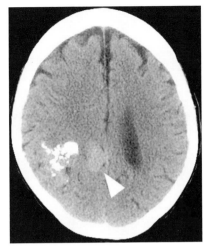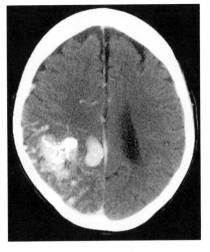

Arteriovenous malformation: mixed density lesion composed of coarse calcification, and faintly hyperdense vessels (arrowhead). Marked enhancement post-contrast.

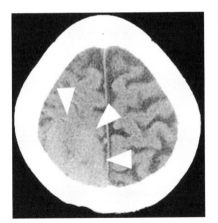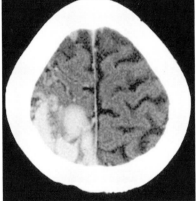

Arteriovenous malformation: large, faintly hyperdense, cortical vessels seen at the right vertex (arrowheads), with marked enhancement post-contrast.

Solitary lesions

Characteristics

- Solitary space-occupying lesions are usually tumours.
  - 30% are secondary tumours from breast, lung or melanoma primary lesions.
  - Metastases tend to be most commonly found in the supratentorial compartment with the exception of those from renal cell carcinoma that tend to be in the posterior fossa.
- Primary tumours (e.g. astrocytoma, glioblastoma multiforme, oligo-dendrogliomas, ependymomas) have a < 50% 5-year survival.
- Frontal lobe masses often present late.
- Other solitary lesions include cerebral abscess, aneurysm, tuberculoma, granuloma or cyst.

Clinical features

- May present with signs of raised intracranial pressure.
- Seizures, with or without a localising aura, are a common first presentation in adults.
- Focal neurology may evolve.
- There may be false localising signs.
- Solitary mass lesions can cause local effects, e.g. proptosis or epistaxis.
- Patients may present with odd behaviour, headache or vomiting.
- The presence of papilloedema is unreliable.
- Clinical presentation may help localise the site of the lesion:
  - *Temporal lobe* – complex partial seizures, hallucinations, déjà vu, taste, smell, dysphasia, field defects, fugue, functional psychosis and hypersexuality.
  - *Frontal lobe* – hemiparesis, seizures, personality change, grasp reflex (unilateral is significant), expressive dysphasia (Broca's area) and anosmia.
  - *Parietal lobe* – hemisensory loss, decreased stereognosis, sensory inattention, dysphasia and Gerstmann's syndrome (finger agnosia, left/right disorientation, dysgraphia, acalculia).
  - *Occipital lobe* – contralateral visual field defects.
  - *Cerebellum* – past pointing, intention tremor, nystagmus, dysdiado-chokinesis and truncal ataxia (worse if eyes open).
  - *Cerebello-pontine angle* – nystagmus, reduced corneal reflex, fifth and seventh cranial nerve palsies, ipsilateral cerebellar signs and ipsilateral deafness.
  - *Mid-brain* – unequal pupils, confabulation, somnolence and an inability to direct the eyes up or down.

Radiological features

- Cerebral masses encompass a spectrum of appearances.
- Lesions may be hypodense, isodense or hyperdense (**see Appendix 1**).
- May be seen due to asymmetry or the presence of oedema and mass effect.
- Calcification may be present.
- Appearance post-contrast is often helpful.

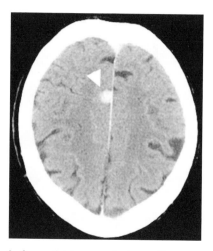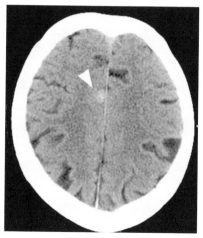

Left parafalcine meningioma: Scans pre- and post-i.v. contrast. The lesion is faintly hyperdense prior to contrast and avidly enhances post-contrast (arrowheads).

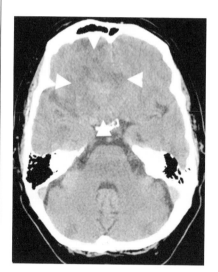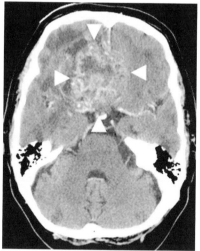

Right frontal glioma. Scans pre- and post-contrast. Subtle heterogeneous, ill-defined mass within the right supra-orbital frontal lobe (arrowheads). Significant enhancement is seen post-contrast, with central non-enhancement, due to necrosis. The peripheral low density relates to vasogenic oedema.

Multiple lesions

Characteristics

- *Neoplastic causes*: Brain metastases are the most common neoplastic intracerebral lesion. They are found in up to 24% of all patients that die from cancer, and represent 20–30% of all brain tumours in adults.
- *Infective causes*: For example, cerebral abscesses, granulomata.
- *Vascular causes*: Multiple lesions of varying age are seen in multi-infarct dementia.
- *Inflammatory causes*: Demyelinating plaques can be seen as multiple low density lesions on CT, predominantly in the periventricular deep white matter.
- *Traumatic causes*: Contusions are frequently multiple after head trauma.

Clinical features

- Depends on the underlying pathology.
- See solitary lesions.

Radiological features

- Contrast is taken up in tumours, inflammatory granulation tissue or areas of damage to the blood–brain barrier. Melanoma and adenocarcinoma metastases may appear hyperdense prior to contrast.
- Calcification in malignant tumours is uncommon but, if present, suggests an adenocarcinoma. Calcification following granulomatous infection in not uncommon.
- Haemorrhage into metastases occurs infrequently, and when present suggests hypervascular tumours such as melanoma or hypernephroma.
- A follow-up CT performed two weeks after a traumatic event makes multiple contusions more conspicuous.

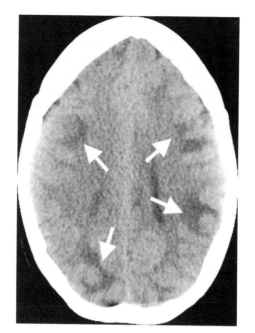

Multiple cerebral metastases. On this unenhanced scan their position is inferred by the associated oedema (arrows).

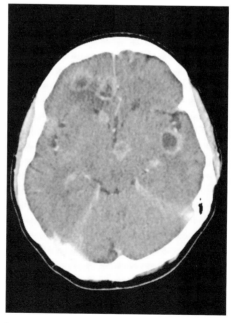

Multiple necrotic ring-enhancing metastases.

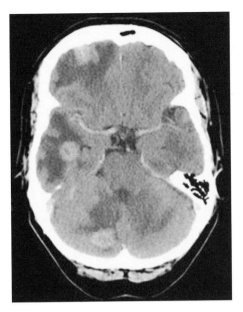

Multiple solid-enhancing metastases with prominent surrounding vasogenic oedema.

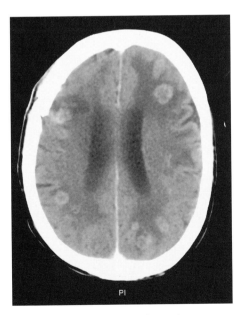

Multiple ring-enhancing tuberculomas.

Self-assessment section

Below are 12 random cases that vary in complexity from easy to difficult. This test is somewhat artificial as no clinical information is given and hence assessment is 'blind'. Formulate a provisional report and compare to the annotated answers at the end.

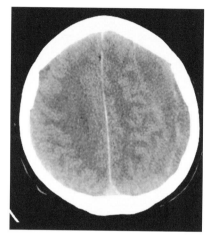

Case 1.

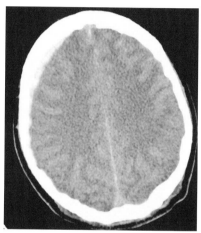

Case 2.

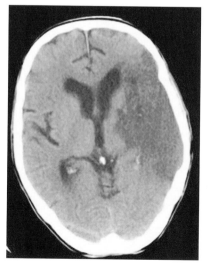

Case 3.

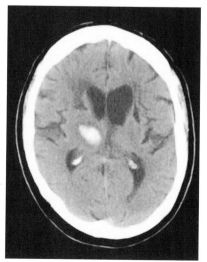

Case 4.

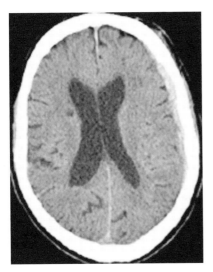

Case 5.

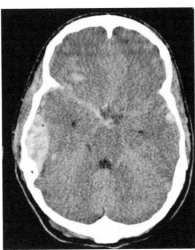

Case 6.

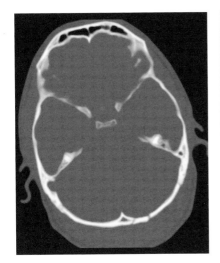

Case 7.

Case 8.

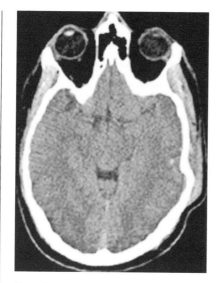

Case 9.

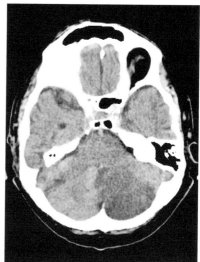

Case 10.

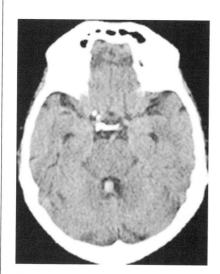

Case 11.

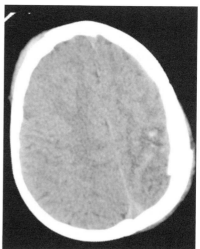

Case 12.

Self Assessment – Answers

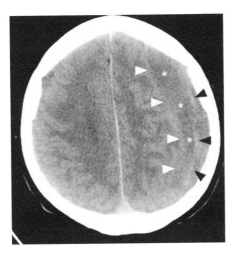

Case 1. A large collection is seen over the left cerebral convexity. This is slightly hypodense to grey matter (asterisk), suggesting that it is somewhat chronic, and exerts mass effect on the adjacent cerebral hemisphere (white arrowheads). Additionally, linear hyperdensity is also seen within the collection (black arrowheads), indicating more acute haemorrhage.
Diagnosis: Acute on chronic subdural haemorrhage.

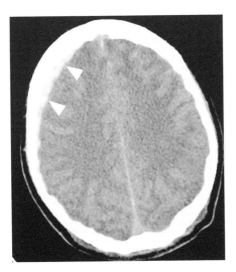

Case 2. A shallow hyperdense collection is seen over the right frontal lobe (arrowheads).
Diagnosis: Acute subdural haemorrhage.

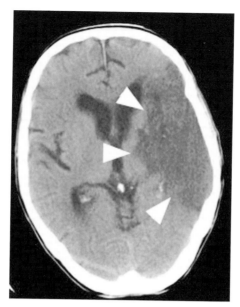

Case 3. Large area of low density, involving both grey and white matter, within the left middle cerebral artery territory (arrowheads). This does not demonstrate haemorrhagic transformation.

Diagnosis: Acute left middle cerebral artery territory infarct.

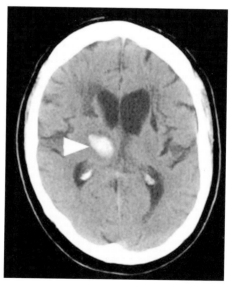

Case 4. Focal area of hyperdensity centred upon the right thalamus and lentiform nucleus (arrowhead).

Diagnosis: Acute parenchymal haemorrhage. This type of haemorrhage has a strong association with uncontrolled hypertension.

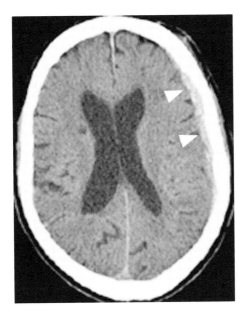

Case 5. A shallow hyperdense collection is seen over the left cerebral convexity (arrowheads).
Diagnosis: Acute subdural haemorrhage.

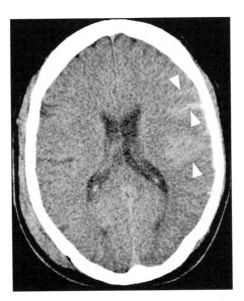

Case 6. Subtle linear hyperdensity is seen outlining several sulci within the left cerebral hemisphere (arrowheads).
Diagnosis: Acute subarachnoid haemorrhage.

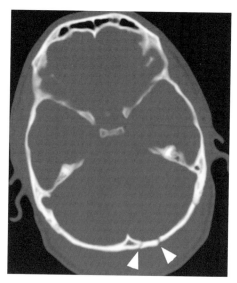

Case 7. Axial scan viewed on 'bone windows', demonstrating sharply marginated defects within the left occipital bone (arrowheads).
Diagnosis: Left occipital fracture.

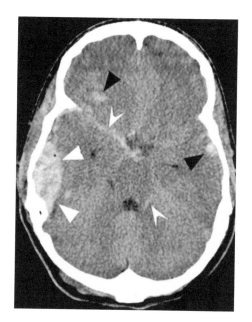

Case 8.
1. Hyperdense biconvex collection over the right temporal lobe (straight white arrowheads).
2. Linear hyperdensity outlining the basal cisterns (curved arrowheads).
3. Focal parenchymal hyperdensity (black arrowheads).
Diagnosis: Acute extradural haemorrhage with additional subarachnoid haemorrhage and parenchymal contusions.

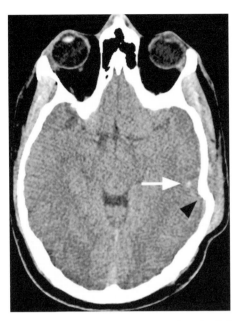

Case 9. Small focal area of hyperdensity seen within the left temporal lobe (arrow), with a small depression in the overlying left temporal bone (arrowhead). This should be assessed formally on bone windows.
Diagnosis: Depressed skull fracture with focal parenchymal contusion.

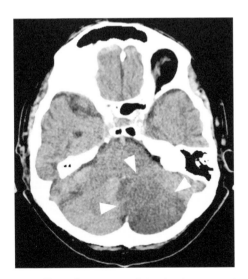

Case 10. Large area of low density, involving both grey and white matter, within the left cerebellar hemisphere (arrowheads). Associated compression of the fourth ventricle due to mass effect.
Diagnosis: Acute left cerebellar infarct.

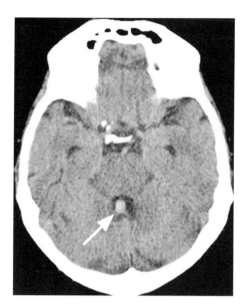

Case 11. Hyperdense focus within the fourth ventricle (arrow).
Diagnosis: Acute intraventricular haemorrhage.

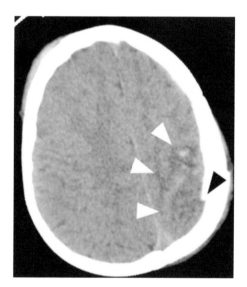

Case 12. Small punctuate and linear areas of hyperdensity seen within the left superior parietal lobe, which is generally of reduced density (white arrowheads). In addition, there is a small 'step' in the inner table of the overlying parietal bone (black arrowhead). This should be formally assessed on bone windows.
Diagnosis: Left superior parietal contusions secondary to a depressed skull fracture.

APPENDICES

APPENDIX I

Differential diagnosis of intracerebral lesions

Calcified intracranial lesions	
Physiological	Choroid plexus, pineal.
Neoplastic	Glioma – 5–10% (20% of astrocytomas). Meningioma – 15% calcify. Metastases – occasionally calcify, particularly colon, breast and osteosarcoma. Craniopharyngioma – 90% calcify in children, 40% in adults. Chordoma – dense calcification in 50% adjacent to the clivus.
Vascular	Aneurysm – 1% calcify. AVMs – 15% calcify. Chronic subdural haematoma – 1–5% calcify. Chronic infarct.
Infective	Abscess – calcification occurs late. Tuberculoma – 1–5% calcify. Usually multiple. Tuberculous meningitis. Cysticercosis.

CT attenuation of cerebral masses (relative to normal brain)

Hyperdense	Isodense	Hypodense
Haematoma < 1 weeks	Haematoma 1–2 weeks	Haematoma >2 weeks
Colloid cyst 50%	Colloid cyst 50%	Cysts: Arachnoid, porencephalic, hydatid
Tuberculoma	Tuberculoma	Tuberculoma
Giant aneurysm	–	Pyogenic abscess
	Neoplasms	
Meningioma 95%	–	–
Primary lymphoma	–	–
Metastases 30%	Metastases 10%	Metastases 30%
Glioma 10%	Glioma 10%	Glioma
Ependymoma	–	–
Medulloblastoma 80%	–	–
Pituitary adenoma 25%	Pituitary adenoma 65%	–
Acoustic neuroma 5%	Acoustic neuroma 95%	–
–	–	Prolactinoma
–	–	Haemangioblastoma
Papilloma	Chordoma	Lipoma
–	Pinealoma	Epidermoid
–	–	Dermoid
Craniopharyngioma (solid)	–	Craniopharyngioma

APPENDIX 2
CT guidelines for head trauma

The National Institute of Clinical Excellence (NICE) Guidelines suggest the following patients with a head injury require CT imaging of the head within 1 hour of the request:

- GCS documented as <13 at any point since the injury.
- GCS 13 or 14 at 2 hours after the injury.
- Focal neurological deficit.
- Clinically suspected open or depressed skull fracture.
- Clinical signs of a basal skull fracture.
- Seizure.
- >1 episode of vomiting.
- Transient loss of consciousness, or amnesia, with any of the following additional features:
  - age ≥ 65yrs.
  - Coagulopathy.
  - On anticoagulation therapy (e.g. Warfarin).

Patients with a transient loss of consciousness, or ante-grade amnesia for greater then 30 minutes, with a dangerous mechanism of injury, should have CT imaging of the head carried out within 8 hours of the injury.

APPENDIX 3

Proposed algorithm for the emergency management of acute stroke

Active management in the initial hours after stroke aims to preserve the ischaemic brain from infarction.

For recognition of suspected stroke, use the FAST test:
- F – Facial movements: New asymmetry
- A – Arm movements: Unilateral arm weakness
- S – Speech: Dysarthria or dysphasia
- T – Telephone 999 in the community. Bleep acute stroke team if yes to any of the above.

Initial management

- Instigate resuscitative measures according to ABC assessment.
- If conscious, sit up.
- Nil by mouth.
- Oxygen to maintain saturation > 95%.
- 100 ml 10% dextrose i.v. if blood glucose < 3 mmols/litre.
- i.v. saline if hypotensive.
- Blood pressure should only be lowered in the acute phase if hypertension is likely to lead to complications (e.g. hypertensive encephalopathy, aortic aneurysm).
- Baseline investigations including ECG, blood and pregnancy test.
- Assess risk of aspiration, using a validated swallowing screening tool.
- Transfer to an Acute Stroke Unit.

Urgent CT imaging of the head should take place for the following patients

- Anticoagulant therapy (e.g. Warfarin).
- Coagulopathies.
- Depressed level of consciousness.
- Papilloedema.
- Neck stiffness.
- Severe headache.
- Progressive or fluctuating neurological symptoms.
- If neurological deficit persists on arrival to hospital, and the onset of symptoms was within 3 hours, **thrombolytic therapy** may be considered. CT must be performed prior to thrombolysis to exclude cerebral haemorrhage.

Exclusion criteria for thrombolytic therapy for acute stroke

- No clear time of symptom onset.
- Decreased level of consciousness.
- Mild clinical deficit or rapidly resolving symptoms.
- Seizure at stroke onset.
- Symptoms suggestive of SAH (even if the CT is normal).
- CT demonstrates any intracranial haemorrhage.
- CT scan showing hypodensity of an evolving infarction, oedema or midline shift.
- CNS aneurysm or AVM.
- BP >185/110 after two attempts to reduce blood pressure.
- Glucose < 2.7 mmol/l or >22.2 mmol/l.
- INR >1.4, APTT >40, or platelet count < 100 000 mm^3.
- Ischaemic stroke, serious head injury, or neurosurgery within the last 3 months.
- Past history of intracranial haemorrhage.
- Pregnancy.
- Standard contraindications for thrombolysis applied to myocardial infarction.

Thrombolysis protocol

- Administer Alteplase 0.9 mg × body weight in kg.
- Give 10% of total dose as a bolus at 1 mg/ml.
- Infuse 90% of total dose at 1 mg/ml over 60 min.

Post-thrombolysis protocol

- Assess GCS hourly for 12 hours.
- BP and pulse every 15 minutes for 2 hours, then every 30 minutes for 6 hours, then hourly for 16 hours.
- Treat BP greater than 185/110.
- Repeat head CT at 24 hours or sooner if neurological deterioration occurs.
- Avoid heparin and antiplatelet agents (including aspirin) until repeat CT at 24 hours has excluded haemorrhage.
- Avoid i.m. injections or unnecessary venous or arterial punctures.
- If clinically significant bleeding occurs, stop the thrombolytic therapy. Perform urgent CT scan, and give fibrinogen (discuss with haematology).
- Give supportive i.v. fluids as necessary.

APPENDIX 4

Information required prior to neurosurgical referral

- Before contacting the neurosurgeon, vital information and an updated clinical evaluation must be collated.
- The following list includes the minimum details that must be immediately available:
  - Referring hospital and named Consultant.
  - Patient demographics with hospital number.
  - Date and time of incident.
  - Time of admission.
  - History of event.
  - Physiological observations.

Time	HR	BP	RR	O$_2$ sat^n	GCS eye	GCS motor	GCS verbal	Right pupil reacts	Right pupil size	Left pupil reacts	Left pupil size
On arrival											
On transfer											

- CT scan/s at referring hospital   Yes   No
- Result of CT scan of head:
- CT scan of neck/chest/abdomen/pelvis/face:
- Other injuries:
- Relevant past medical history:
- Allergies:
- Drug history:
- Last ingestion:
- Interventions: Airway: Guedel   ETT
                 Breathing: Spontaneous   IPPV
                 Circulation: Fluids   Urinary catheter
- Drugs given:
- Tetanus:
- Blood test results:
- X-match:
- Arterial blood gas:
- Urinalysis:
- Next of kin contact details: Notified: Yes   No
- Medical escort:

- Documentation for transfer: medical notes/Observation chart/ Radiographs
- Receiving neurosurgeon:
- ETA: